HOW TO Name a Baby*

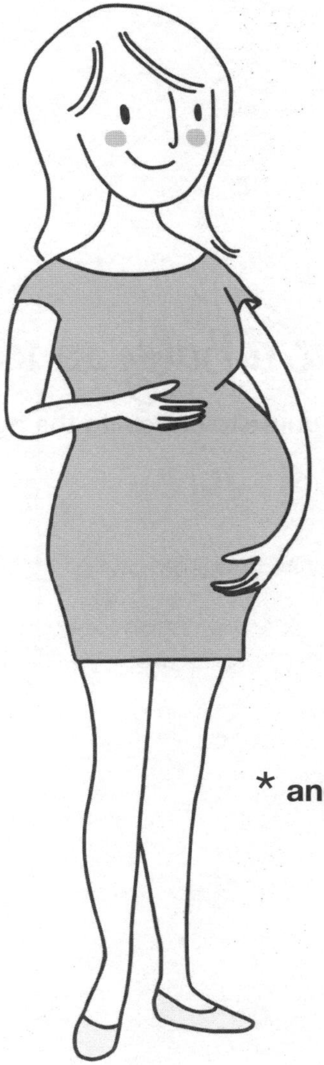

* and Get it Right

Sophie Shaw

How To *Name a Baby* ...and Get it Right

The essential pocket guide to choosing the right name for your baby

Created by Sophie Shaw

ISBN: 978-1-912155-27-9

BELL & MACKENZIE
PUBLISHING LIMITED
www.bellmackenzie.com

Contents

* Tips To Help You Name Your Baby 5

* Girls Names A - F 10
  G - L 30
  M - R 48
  S - Z 61

* Boys Names A - F 74
  G - L 95
  M - R 113
  S - Z 126

* 100 Popular Girls Names 137

* 100 Popular Boys Names 141

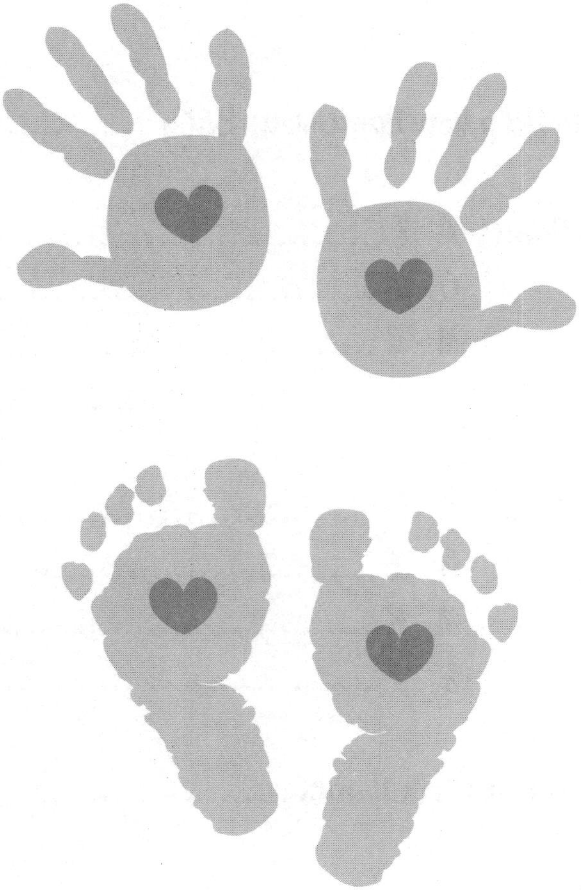

HOW TO Name a Baby

...and Get it Right

Ok so it's time to name your baby. In this book you'll find 5000 baby names from around the world along with meanings, derivatives and a list of some of the most popular UK girls and boys names.

Choosing a name can be really easy. Many parents ease through the process... but not everyone! For others, choosing a name for your baby can be a frustrating and agonising process which doesn't feel like a joy and hangs over you like a cloud. Fear not. Here are some simple tips to help you name your baby...and get it right!

Inspiration

This might sound obvious, but try really opening your eyes and ears to the world around you. Listen to the names you hear in conversation or the names you read in books or see in films. Think about your heroes whether that's a character in a book or the subject of a song. Write down any interesting names you hear which you can browse through from time to time until something clicks into place.

Popular Names

Some parents prefer not to choose a name that's already in the top 10. Others love that the name is popular. It's all about personal preference.
You may however want to avoid choosing the same baby name as high-profile celebrities. Otherwise, you may be constantly asked if this influenced your name choice – unless of course you are happy with that.

Standing Out From the Crowd

Do you want your child to blend in or stand out?
Be careful here. An unusual name might be great when your child is little and they are happy to be the centre of attention. But will they thank you when they are in their awkward teenage years? Maybe. Maybe not.
Remember the name you give them is not for you. It's for your baby. Something they will carry all their lives.

Surnames & Middle Names

Think about how the names you like work with your child's surname. The final choice has got to work as a complete name. Not just as a first name. Lots of people also give their child a middle name. If you have two names you can't decide on consider using them both. Some people even use multiple middle names that can create a really lovely name combination.

Many people however dislike their middle names, as they are rarely used and so often feel alien to them. So here's an idea... don't give your child a middle name. Let them choose one for themselves when they are older and give them some ownership of their identity.

Unfortunate Word Games

If you do decide to choose a combination of names check that your baby's initials don't spell out an unfortunate word. Take this name for example, **P**eter **I**an **G**oldsmith. No child wants to be a pig!

Nicknames

Think about shortened and lengthened versions of the name you chose. You can't stop your little one's friends altering his or her name. So think about whether you are going to be happy with the potential nicknames.

Connotations

What you think of a name is often coloured by your own life experiences. Your partner might love a name but it might remind you of a girl you disliked in school or an ex-boyfriend you don't want to think about. Try to leave the past behind. Your baby is a brand new start. Look ahead not behind.

Don't let the perfect name pass you by because of the past. Everything will fade into insignificance as soon as you name your baby.

Everyone Grows up

Remember your baby is going to be an adult one day. It's hard to imagine at this moment but it is going to happen so make sure that a cute baby name is going to work for them all their lives.

Spelling

An usual spelling or pronunciation of a name is your choice. It can be a drag if it causes confusion and your child might grow tired of correcting people when they misspell their name or can't pronounce it. Other children embrace it and over the years it can be a source of conversation as well as a great icebreaker.

Keep It To Yourself

Everyone loves to have an opinion. That might be great for you… but it might not. Consider keeping the name to yourselves until you are really sure about it. Grandparents love to push back on unfamiliar names - remember they will be putting all their life experiences into their opinions just like you did. Don't be surprised if everyone doesn't love it straight away. Remember they might need time to get used to it.

If you want to avoid any unwelcome, well-intentioned advice from friends and family don't tell anybody the baby's name until it is born. Then introduce your baby, and their name, to your family for this first time.

Good luck!

Girls

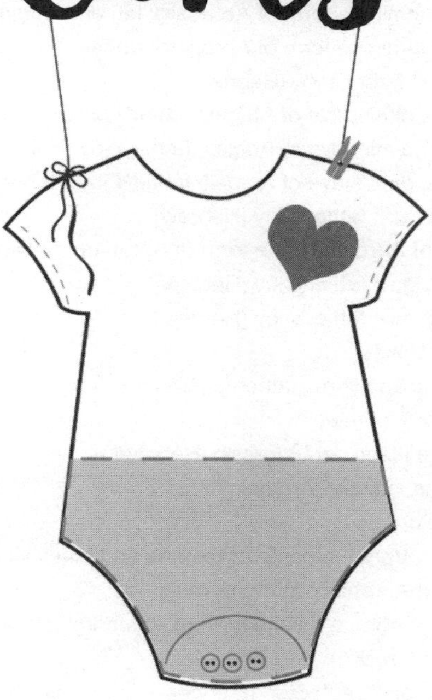

A

Aaliyah	Feminine form of Aali/Ali; lofty, sublime [Arabic]
Aaren	Feminine form of Aaron; high; exalted [Hebrew]
Abagael	Variant of Abigail; father's joy [Hebrew]
Abalene	Variant of Abilene, Biblical place name; grass [Hebrew]
Abalina	Variant of Abilene, Biblical place name; grass [Hebrew]
Abame	Variant of Abra, feminine form of Abraham; father of multitudes [Hebrew]
Abaranne	Variant of Abra, feminine form of Abraham; father of multitudes [Hebrew]
Abbagail	Variant of Abigail; father's joy [Hebrew]
Abbe	Variant of Abbie, diminutive of Abigail; father's joy [Hebrew]
Abbea	Variant of Abbie, diminutive of Abigail; father's joy [Hebrew]
Abbee	Variant of Abbie, diminutive of Abigail; father's joy [Hebrew]
Abbie	Diminutive of Abigail; father's joy [Hebrew]
Abbrienna	Elaborate form of Abra, feminine form of Abraham; father of multitudes
Abby	Diminutive of Abigail; father's joy [Hebrew]
Abi	Diminutive of Abigail; father's joy [Hebrew]
Abigail	Father's joy [Hebrew]
Abijah	Variant of Abijah; God is my father [Hebrew]
Abijah	God is my father [Hebrew]
Abilene	From the Biblical place name; grass [Hebrew]
Abitha	Variant of Tabitha; gazelle [Aramaic]
Abla	Full-figure [Arabic]
Abony	Variant of Ebony; from the name of the tree and black wood [Egyptian]
Abra	Feminine form of Abraham; father of multitudes
Abrea	Elaborate form of Abra, feminine form of Abraham; father of multitudes
Abrial	Open; protected [French]
Abrilla	Variant of Abrial; pen; protected [French]
Acacia	From the name of the tree
Acadia	Idyllic place [Greek]
Acantha	Thorn [Greek]
Acasia	Variant of Acacia; from the name of the tree
Achanti	Variant of Ashanti; from the African place name
Acie	Diminutive of Acacia; from the name of the tree
Ada	Noble one [Old German]
Adabella	Elaborate form of Ada; noble one [Old German]
Adabelle	Elaborate form of Ada; noble one [Old German]
Adair	From the surname; derived from Edgar; wealthy spearsman [Old English]

Adalaide	Variant of Adelaide; noble; kind [Old German]
Adalia	Noble one [Hebrew]
Adalyn	Variant of Adeline; noble; diminutive of Adele
Adamina	Feminine form of Adam; man [Hebrew]
Adara	Virgin; noble; exalted [Arabic & Hebrew]
Addie	Diminutive of Adelaide, Adaline or other names beginning with Ad-
Addison	From the surname; “son of Adam”
Addisyn	Variant of Addison; from the surname;”son of Adam”
Adela	Noble one
Adelaide	Noble; kind [Old German]
Adele	Noble one [French]
Adelfia	Variant of Adelpha; beloved sister [Greek]
Adelina	Variant of Adeline; noble; diminutive of Adele
Adeline	Noble, diminutive of Adele
Adeliza	Variant of Adelaide; noble; kind [Old German]
Adelpha	Beloved sister [Greek]
Adelphia	Variant of Adelpha; beloved sister [Greek]
Adelyn	Variant of Adeline; noble; diminutive of Adele
Adhara	Virgins [Arabic]
Adina	Variant of Edina; wealthy one [Old English]
Adira	Strong [Hebrew]
Adora	Adored; loved [Latin]
Adriana	Dark; from Adria [Latin, Italian]
Aerial	Variant of Ariel; lion of God [Hebrew]
Aeron	From a Celtic goddess of war [Welsh]
Aeronwy	Elaborate form of Aeron; from a Celtic goddess of war [Welsh]
Aeronwyn	Elaborate form of Aeron; from a Celtic goddess of war [Welsh]
Affrika	Variant of Africa; from the continent of Africa
Afra	Diminutive of Africa; from the continent of Africa
Africa	From the continent of Africa
Afrodite	Variant of Aphrodite; name of the goddess of love [Greek]
Agatha	Good; kind [Greek]
Agata	European form of Agatha; good; kind [Greek]
Aggie	Diminutive of Agatha or Agnes
Agnes	Pure one [Greek]
Aida	Helpful one [Latin]
Aideen	Little fire [Irish]
Aileen	Light bearer
Ailis	Irish form of Alice; noble one; variant of Adelaide [Greek]
Ailsa	From Ailsa Craig, a rocky island in the Firth of Clyde
Aimee	Variant of Amy; Beloved one [Old French]
Ainsley	From surname/placename; from the woodland hermitage [Old English]
Aisha	Living; prosperous [Arabic]
Alaina	Variant of Alana; beautiful child; little rock [Irish]

Alana	Beautiful child; little rock [Irish]
Alani	Orange tree [Hawaiian]
Alanis	Precious; awakening [Old German]
Alannah	Little rock; precious; variant of Alana
Alba	White [Latin]
Alberta	Noble one; bright
Alda	Prosperous one [Old German]
Aleah	Variant of Aaliya; lofty, sublime [Arabic]
Alessandra	Italian variant of Alexandra; the defender [Greek]
Aletha	Variant of Alethea; truth [Greek]
Alethea	Truth [Greek]
Alexa	A derivative of Alexandra; the defender [Greek]
Alexandra	The defender [Greek]
Alexia	A derivative of Alexandra; the defender [Greek]
Alexia	A derivative of Alexandra; the defender [Greek]
Alexis	A derivative of Alexandra; the defender [Greek]
Alexus	Variant of Alexis; the defender [Greek]
Ali	Diminutive of Alexandra, Alexis, Alison etc
Alice	Noble one; variant of Adelaide [Greek]
Alicia	A derivative of Alice; noble one [Greek]
Alison	Diminutive of Alice; noble one [Old German]
Alix	Noble one [Old German]
Allegra	Lively [Italian]
Ally	Noble and bright one [Old German]
Alma	Good one; nourishing [Celtic; Latin]
Aloisia	Feminine form of Aloysius; famous in battle [Old German]
Alouetta	From alouette; lark [French]
Alva	White one [Latin]
Alvina	Elf friend [Old English]
Alys	Noble; variant of Alys
Alyson	Noble; diminutive of Alys
Alyssa	Variant of Alice; noble one [Greek]
Amabel	Loveable one [Latin]
Amanda	Worthy of love [Latin]
Amber	The sky [Sanskrit]; or from the gemstone
Ambrosia	Feminine form of Ambrose; immortal [Greek]
Amelia	Industrious, striving [Old German]
Amelie	Variant of Amelia; industrious; striving [Old German]
Amethyst	Protector
Amity	Frienliness; friendship
Amy	Beloved one [Old French]
An	Peace [Chinese]
Anastasia	Resurrection [Greek]
Andrea	Strength; manly [Greek]

Angel	Angelic one; messenger [Greek]
Angela	Angelic one [Greek]
Angelica	Angelic one [Latin]
Angelina	Diminutive of Angela
Anita	Diminutive of Anna; favour; grace
Ann	Variant of Anne; grace, favour [Hebrew]
Anna	Favour; grace [Hebrew]
Annabel	Loving; loveable
Anne	Variant of Hannah; grace [Hebrew]
Annette	French diminutive of Anne; faour, grace [Hebrew]
Annie	Variant of Anna and Anne; grace
Annis	Form of Agnes; pure one
Annora	Variant of Honor/Honour; the virtue, honour
Annushka	Russian diminutive of Anna; grace; favour [Hebrew]
Anouk	Dutch variant of Anna; grace; favour [Hebrew]
Antonia	Beautiful; priceless [Latin]
Anwen	Fair; beautiful [Welsh]
Aphra	Variant of Afra, diminutive of Africa; from the continent of Africa
Aphrodite	Name of the goddess of love [Greek]
April	To open / blossom [Latin]
Arabella	Variant of Annabel; loving, lovable
Araminta	Aminta + Arabella; prayer and protection
Arcadia	Place of ideal peace & contentment; from Arcadia in the Greek Peleponese
Arden	High [Celtic
Aretha	Virtue [Greek]
Aria	Song [Italian]
Ariadne	Most holy [Greek]
Arianna	Latin form of Ariadne; most holy [Greek]
Arianne	French form of Ariadne; most holy [Greek]
Ariel	Lion of God [Hebrew]
Ariella	Form of Ariel; lion of God [Hebrew]
Arienne	Variant of Arianne, French form of Ariadne; most holy [Greek]
Arlene	Unknown meaning
Arlo	Possibly from the Irish place name Aherlow; between two high lands [Irish]
Artemesia	Gift of Artemis [Greek]
Ash	From the name of the tree. Or diminutive of Ashleigh, Ashlyn etc.
Ashanti	From the Afriacna place name
Ashleigh	Ash meadow [Old English]
Ashley	Variant of Ashleigh; ash medow
Ashlyn	Combination of Ashleigh and Lyn
Astra	Star [Greek]
Astrid	Beautiful Goddess [Old Norse]
Aubrey	Feminine variant of Alberich; powerful [old German]
Auden	From the surname; old friend [Old German]

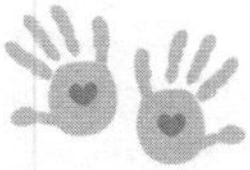

Audra Variant of Audrey; noble; strength [old English]
Audrey Noble; strength [old English]
Augusta Great [Latin]
Aura Aura; atmosphere
Aurelie Golden [Latin]
Aurora Dawn [Latin]
Autumn Autumn
Ava Variant of Eve; to breathe
Avalon Island of Apples [Celtic]
Aveline Diminutive of Avila; desired [Old German]
Avery From the surname; powerful [old German]
Avila Desired [Old German]
Avis Desired [Old German]
Aviva The season of spring [Hebrew]
Avril French form of April; to open/ blossom [Latin]
Azaria God has helped [Hebrew]
Azariah Variant of Azaria; God has helped [Hebrew]

B

Bab Diminutive of Barbara; foreign [Greek]
Babette Diminutive of Barbara; foreign [Greek]
Baboshka Butterfly [Russian]
Babs Diminutive of Barbara; foreign [Greek]
Bae Variant of Bay; berry [Latin]
Baha Variant of Baja; from Baja, Spain [Spanish]
Baileigh Varient of Bailey; bailiff [Old English]
Bailey Bailiff [Old English]
Bailie Variant of Bailey; bailiff [Old English]
Bailor Variant of Baylor; horse trainer [Old English]
Baja From Baja, Spain [Spanish]
Ballou From the surname; from Ballou [French]
Balou Variant of Ballou; from the surname; from Ballou [French]
Banjo From the name of the musical instrument
Bao Creative [Chinese]
Baptista Baptised one [Latin]
Barbara Foreign [Greek]
Barbra Variant of Barbara; foreign [Greek]
Barcelona From the name of the Spanish city

Bardot	From the surname [French]
Barett	From the surname; quarrelsome [Old English]; bear strength [Old German]
Barrett	From the surname; quarrelsome [Old English]; bear strength [Old German]
Barri	Feminine form of Barry; head [Gaelic]
Basilia	Feminine form of Basil; king [Greek]
Basilie	Variant of Basilia, a feminine form of Basil; king [Greek]
Bathseva	Variant of Bathsheba; daughter of an oath [Hebrew]
Bathsheba	Daughter of an oath [Hebrew]
Bay	Berry [Latin]
Baylor	Horse trainer [Old English]
Bea	Diminutive of Beatrix; traveller [Latin]
Beata	Blessed [Latin]
Beate	Blessed [Latin]
Beatrice	Form of Beatrix; traveller [Latin]
Beatrix	Traveller [Latin]
Beckie	Diminutive of Rebecca; join [Hebrew]
Becky	Diminutive of Rebecca; join [Hebrew]
Bekka	Diminutive of Rebecca; join [Hebrew]
Belinda	Beautiful and soft; bright serpent [Italian; old German]
Bella	Beautiful [Italian]; or diminutive of Isabella etc.
Belladonna	From the name of the poisonous flower; nightshade
Ballamy	From the surname; beautiful friend [Old French]
Belle	Beautiful [French]; or diminutive of Isabelle etc.
Belva	Beautiful view [French]
Benazir	Incomparable; unique {Pakistani]
Benedetta	Blessed [Latin]
Benedicta	Blessed [Latin]
Berenice	Bringing victory [Greek]
Bernadette	Brave; strong as a bear [[old German]
Bernadine	Brave; strong as a bear [[old German]
Bernice	Diminutive of Berenice; bringing victory [Latin]
Bernie	Diminutive of Bernadette, Bernice etc.
Berri	Variant of Berry; berry
Berrill	Variant of Beryl; from the precious stone
Berry	Berry
Bertha	Bright; famous [old German]
Bertie	Diminutive of Bertha, Roberta and other names containing -bert-
Beryl	From the precious stone [Sanskritt]
Bess	Diminutive of Elizabeth; oath of God
Beth	Diminutive of Elizabeth; or diminutive of Bethany; house of figs
Bethan	Diminutive of Elizabeth or of Bethany
Bethany	From the town; house of figs [Hebrew]
Betony	The herb betony
Betsy	Diminutive of Elizabeth; oath of God

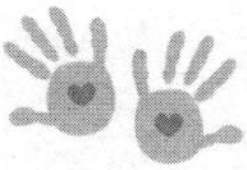

Bette	Diminutive of Elizabeth; oath of God
Betty	Diminutive of Elizabeth; oath of God
Beulah	Married [Hebrew]
Beverley	From the English city; beaver stream
Beverly	Variant of Beverley; beaver stream
Bianca	White [Italian]
Biancha	Variant of Bianca; white [Italian]
Bianka	Variant of Bianca; white [Italian]
Biddy	Diminutive of Bridget; exalted one [Irish]
Bijou	Jewel [French]
Billie	Diminutive of Wilhelmina; resolute protector
Birdie	Little bird; bird-like
Blanche	White/fair [French]
Blossom	Blossom
Blythe	Formed frm surname Blythe; cheerful [old English]
Bobbi	Diminutive of Roberta; bright fame
Bobbie	Diminutive of Roberta; bright fame
Bobby	Diminutive of Roberta; bright fame
Bobette	Diminutive of Roberta; bright fame
Bobina	Diminutive of Roberta; bright fame
Bonita	Pretty [Spanish]
Bonnie	Pretty [Old French/Scots]
Brandi	Variant of Brandy; alcholic drink
Brandy	Alcoholic drink
Branwen	Blessed raven [Welsh]
Breanna	Variant of Brianna; high, noble [Celtic]
Breanne	Variant of Brianna; high, noble [Celtic]
Brenda	Sword [Old Norse]
Brenna	Variant of Brenda; sword [Old Norse]
Brianna	High; noble [Celtic]
Brianne	Variant of Brianna; high, noble [Celtic]
Briar	Briar; thorny plant
Bridget	Exalted one [Irish]
Brighton	From the name of the English town; bright town
Briony	Briony, vine
Britannia	Britain [Latin]
Brittany	Brittany in France
Brittney	Variant of Brittany
Bronwen	White breast [Welsh]
Brook	From the surname; one who lives near a brook
Brooke	Variant of Brook; one who lives near a brook
Brooklyn	Area of New York City
Bryn	Hill [Welsh]
Buffy	Diminutive of Elizabeth; oath of God

Bunny	Diminutive of Berenice; traveller [Latin]
Butterfly	Butterfly

C

Cachet	Prestigious [French]
Caddie	Diminutive of Cadence; rhtyhm; inflection
Cadeau	Gift [French]
Cadence	Rhythm; inflection
Cadenza	Italian variant of Cadence; from the musical term
Cadia	Diminutive of Arcadia; place of ideal peace and contentment
Cadiz	From the name of the Spanish city
Cai	Feminine form of Kai; sea [Hawaiian]. Or feminine [Vietnamese
Caileen	Variant of Cailin; girl [Irish]
Cailin	Girl [Irish]
Caitlin	Irish form of Kathleen/Katherine; pure [Greek]
Caitlyn	Variant of Caitlin; pure [Greek]
Cala	Castle; fortress [Arabic]
Calais	From the name of the French port
Calder	From the surname; rocky water [Old English]
Caledonia	Scotland [Latin]
Calico	From the name of the cotton fabric
Calida	Heated [Spanish]
Calinda	Variant of Calida; heated [Spanish]
Calipso	Variant of Calypso; she who hides [Greek]
Calista	Most beautiful [Greek]
Calixta	Variant of Calista; most beautiful [Greek]
Calla	Type of lily; beautiful [Greek]
Callie	Diminutive of Caroline; warrior [Old German]
Calliope	Beautiful voice [Greek]; from the name of the Greek goddess
Calvina	Feminine form of Calvin; from the French surname Chauvin; bald [Latin]
Calypso	She who hides [Greek]
Camellia	From the flowering shrub
Cameron	From the surname; crooked nose [Scottish]
Camilla	Unblemished virgin; ceremonial attendant [Latin]
Camille	Variant of Camilla; ublemished virgin; ceremonial attendant [Latin]
Cammy	Diminutive of Camilla; ublemished virgin; ceremonial attendant [Latin]
Camryn	Variant of Cameron; crooked nose [Scottish]
Candace	Queen mother [Cushitic]
Candi	Variant of Candy; sweet; or diminutive of Candace

Candice	Variant of Candace; queen mother [Cushitic]
Candida	White [Latin]
Candra	Variant of Chandra; goddess of the moon [Hindi]
Candy	Sweet; or diminutive of Candace
Canyon	Canyon
Capria	Variant of Caprice; impulsive [Italian]
Caprice	Impulsive [Italian]
Cara	Beloved [Italian]
Caren	Variant of Karen; pure
Carey	From the surname; black
Carina	Form of Cara; beloved [Italian]
Carla	Warrior [Old German]
Carlene	Dimintive of Carla; warrior [Old German]
Carlita	Variant of Carlotta; Spanish diminutive of Charles; warrior [Old German]
Carlotta	Spanish feminine diminutive of Charles; warrior [Old German]
Carly	Variant of Carla; warrior [Old German]
Carlyn	Variant of Caroline; warrior [Old German]
Carmel	Garden [Hebrew]
Carmelita	Diminutive of Carmel; garden [Hebrew]
Carmella	Variant of Carmel; garden [Hebrew]
Carmen	Song [Latin] Or variant of Carmel; garden [Hebrew]
Carol	Diminutive of Caroline; warrior [Old German]. Or hymn/song
Carolina	Variant of Caroline; warrior [Old German]
Caroline	Warrior [Old German]
Carolyn	Variant of Caroline; warrior [Old German]
Carrie	Diminutive of Caroline; warrior [old German]
Casey	From the surname; vigilant [Irish]
Cass	Diminutive of Cassandra, Cassidy etc
Cassandra	Excell; shine [Greek]
Cassia	Feminine form of Cassius; vain; empty [Latin]
Cassidy	From the surname; curly-haired [Irish]
Cassie	Diminutive of Cassandra, Cassidy etc
Cat	Diminutive of Catherine/Katherine; pure [Greek]
Cate	Variant of Kate, diminutive of Catherine/Katherine; pure [Greek]
Catharine	Variant of Catherine/Katherine; pure [Greek]
Catherine	Variant of Katherine; pure [Greek]
Cathleen	Variant of Kathleen; pure [Greek]
Cathryn	Variant of Catherine/Katherine; pure [Greek]
Cathy	Diminutive of Catherine/Katherine; pure [Greek]
Catriona	Gaelic form of Catherine/Katherine; pure [Greek]
Cecelia	Variant of Cecilia; blind [Latin]
Cecilia	Blind [Latin]
Cecily	English form of Cecilia; blind [Latin]
Celandine	From the flower

Celeste	Heavenly [Latin]
Celestine	English form of Celeste; heavenly [Latin]
Celia	Heaven [Latin]. Or diminutive of Cecila; blind [Latin]
Celine	Heavenly [Latin]
Cenobia	Spanish form of Zenobia; force of Zeus [Greek]
Ceres	Roman goddess of the harvest {Latin]
Ceridwen	Beautiful as a poem [Welsh]
Cerise	Cherry; or its colour [French]
Cerissa	Variant of Cerise; cherry; or its colour [French]
Cerys	Love [Welsh]
Chandra	Goddess of the moon [Hindi]
Chanel	From the surname; pipe [French]; influenced by designer Coco Chanel
Channelle	Variant of Chanel; pipe [French]
Channing	From the surname; little wolf cub
Chantal	Stony; song [French]
Chanté	Sung [French]
Chantel	Variant of Chantal; stony; song [French]
Charis	Grace; kindness [Greek]
Charisma	Personal magnetism; grace [Greek]
Charissa	Form of Charis; grace; kindness [Greek]
Charisse	From the French surname; grace; kindness [Greek]
Charity	Generous love [Greek]
Charla	Feminine form of Charles; warrior [Old German]
Charlene	Feminine diminutive of Charles; warrior [Old German]
Charley	Diminutive of Charlotte, a feminine diminutive of Charles; warrior [old German]
Charlie	Diminutive of Charlotte, a feminine diminutive of Charles; warrior [old German]
Charlotte	Feminine diminutive of Charles; warrior [Old German]
Charmaine	Possibly a form of Charmion; delight [Greek]
Chasity	Variant of Chastity; pure [Latin]
Chastity	Pure [Latin]
Chelle	Diminutive of Michelle; who is like God? [Hebrew]
Chelsea	Area of London
Chelsey	Variant of Chelsea; area of London
Cher	Diminutive of Cherie or Cheryl; darling [French]
Cheri	Variant of Cherie; darling [French]
Cherisse	Variant of Charisse; grace; kindness [Greek]
Cherie	Darling [French]
Cherilyn	Cheryl (darling) + -lyn
Cherish	To treasure
Cherry	From the fruit; or diminutive of Charity
Cherryl	Variant of Cheryl; darling [French]
Cheryl	Form of Cherie; darling [French]
Cheyanne	Variant of Cheyenne; from the Native American trieb; red speakers
Cheyenne	From the Native American people; red speakers [Dakota/Native American]

China	From the country
Chloe	Green shoot [Greek]
Chris	Diminutive of Christine etc; Christian
Chrissie	Diminutive of Christine etc; Christian
Chrissy	Diminutive of Christine etc; Christian
Christa	Diminutive of Christine etc; Christian
Christabel	Beautiful Christian
Christabelle	Variant of Christabel; beautiful Christian
Christal	Variant of Crystal
Christi	Diminutive of Christine etc; Christian
Christiana	Latin form of Christine; Christian
Christianne	Variant of Christiana; Christian
Christina	Variant of Christine; Christian
Christine	Christian
Christmas	From the Christian festival
Chrystal	Variant of Crystal
Chyna	Variant of China; from the name of the country
Ciara	Variant of Sierra; mountain range [Spanish]. Or black [Irish]
Cicely	Variant of Cecily; blind [Latin]
Cindi	Diminutive of Cynthia; woman of Kynthos [Greek]
Cindy	Diminutive of Cynthia; woman of Kynthos [Greek]
Circe	Bird [Greek]
Cissy	Variant of Sissy; diminutive of Cecilia, Frances etc
Claire	Variant of Clara; clear; famous [Latin]
Clara	Clear; famous [Latin]
Clare	Variant of Claire/Clara; clear; famous [Latin]
Clarette	Diminutive of Clara; clear; famous [Latin]
Claribel	Clear + beautiful [Latin + French]
Clarice	Variant of Clara; clear; famous [Latin]
Clarinda	Form of Clara; clear; famous [Latin]
Clarissa	Variant of Clarisse/Clara; clear; famous [Latin]
Claude	Lame [Latin]
Claudia	Variant of Claude; lame [Latin]
Clemence	Merciful [Latin]
Clementina	Spanish form of Clemence; merciful [Latin]
Clementine	French variant of Clemence; merciful [Latin]
Cleo	Diminutive of Cleopatra; glory of the father [Greek]
Clotilda	English form of Clotilde; famed in battle {Old German]
Clover	From the wild flower
Coby	Feminine diminutive of Jacob; supplanter [Hebrew]
Cody	From the Irish surname; helpful [Irish]
Coleen	Variant of Colleen; girl [Irish]
Colleen	Girl [Irish]
Connie	Diminutive of Constance; steadfast

Constance Steadfast; constant
Constantine Variant of Constance; steadfast; constant
Cora Maiden [Greek]
Coral From the undersea deposit
Cordelia Daughter of the sea; heart [Celtic]
Coretta Diminutive of Cora; maiden [Greek]
Corey From the surname; hollow dweller; spear
Cori From the surname Corey; hollow dweller; spear
Corina Variant of Corinna; maiden [Greek]
Corinna Maiden [Greek]
Corinne French form of Corinna; maiden [Greek]
Cornelia Feminine form of Cornelius; of the horn [Latin]
Courtney From the surname; short nose [Norman French]
Cressida Golden [Greek]
Crystal Cut glass; ice [Greek]
Cybill Variant of Sibyl; prophetess [Greek]
Cynthia Woman from Kynthos [Greek]
Cyra Feminine form of Cyrus; lord [Greek]. Or sun [Persian]

D

Dacey From the south [Irish]
Daci Variant of Dacey; from the south [Irish]
Dacia From the name of the Roman province in eastern Europe
Dacie Variant of Candace; queen mother [Cushitic]. From the south [Irish]
Dagmar Dane's joy [Old Norse]
Dagna Variant of Dagmar; Dane's joy [Norse]
Dahlia From the flower
Daisy From the flower
Dakota Friends [Dakota/Native American]
Dale From the surname; person living in a dale/valley
Dalicia Variant of Delicia; delicious; delight [Latin]
Dalila Sign from the gods [Swahili]. Or of Delilah; delicate; languishing [Hebrew]
Dalili Sign from the gods [Swahili]
Damania Feminine form of Damian; tame; dometicated [Greek]
Damica Open; friendly [French]
Dana From the surname; Dane; from Denmark. Or Celtic goddess Danu/Dana
Dani Diminutive of Danielle; God is my judge [Hebrew]
Danica Morning star [Slavic]

Daniella	Variant of Danielle; God is my judge [Hebrew]
Danielle	God is my judge [Hebrew]
Danika	Variant of Danica; morning star [Slavic]
Danita	Diminutive of Danielle; God is my judge [Hebrew]
Danna	God is my judge [Hebrew]
Danni	Variant of Dani, diminutive of Danielle; God is my judge [Hebrew]
Daphne	Laurel [Greek]
Darby	From the surname; town of deer [Old Norse]
Darcie	Variant of Darcy; from the surname; coming from town of Arcy,France
Darcy	From the surname; coming from town of Arcy, France
Daria	Possesses; rich/kingly [Persian, Greek]
Darla	Diminutive of Darlene; darling
Darlene	Darling
Davena	Variant of Davina; feminine form of David; beloved [Hebrew
Davina	Feminine form of David; beloved [Hebrew]
Dawn	Dawn of morning
Dawna	Elaborate form of Dawn; dawn of morning
Dawne	Variant of Dawn; dawn of morning
Day	Day
Daya	Elaborate form of Day; day
Dayna	Variant of Dana; from the surname Dane. Or Celtic goddess Danu/Dana
Deana	Variant of Deanna/Dianna; divine [Indo-European]
Deanna	Variant of Dianna; divine [Indo-European]
Deanne	Variant of Deanna/Dianna; divine [Indo-European]
Deb	Diminutive of Deborah; bee [Hebrew]
Debbi	Diminutive of Deborah; bee [Hebrew]
Debbie	Diminutive of Deborah; bee [Hebrew]
Deborah	Bee [Hebrew]
Debra	Variant of Deborah; bee [Hebrew]
Dee	Shortened form of names beginning with D
Deena	Variant of Deanna/Dianna; divine [Indo-European]
Deeva	Variant of Deva; from the name of the Hindu moon goddess [Hindi]
Deidra	Variant of Deirdre; unknown; woman [Celtic]
Deirdre	Unknown; woman [Celtic]
Delaney	From the surname; from the alder grove [Norman French]
Delfina	Variant of Delphia; from Delphi; womb [Greek]
Delia	Of Delos [Greek]
Delice	Variant of Delicia; delicious; delight [Latin]
Delicia	Delicious; delight [Latin]
Delilah	Delicate; languishing [Hebrew]
Dell	From the surname; living in a dell/valley
Della	Diminutive of Adela or Adelaide; noble or noble and kind
Delma	Diminutive of Fidelma; good; beauty [Celtic]; faithful [Latin]
Delora	Variant of Dolores; sorrow [Spanish]

Delores	Variant of Dolores; sorrow [Spanish]
Delphia	From Delphi; womb [Greek]
Delphine	French form of Delphia; from Dephi; womb [Greek]
Delta	Greek letter; river delta
Demelza	From Cornish place name; Maeldaf's fort
Demetra	Variant of Demetria; earth mother [Greek]
Demetria	Earth mother [Greek]
Demi	Half [French]. Or diminutive of Demetria; earth mother [Greek]
Demica	Variant of Damica; open; friendly [French]
Denice	Variant of Denise; god from Nysa [Greek]
Denise	God from Nysa [Greek]
Deona	Variant of Dionne; goddess [Greek]. Or of Deanna; divine [Indo-European]
Deonne	Variant of Dionne; goddess [Greek]
Desirée	Desired [French]
Despina	Lady [Greek]
Destini	Variant of Destiny; fate; destiny
Destiny	Fate; destiny
Destrey	Variant of Destry; war horse [French
Destry	War horse [French]
Deva	From the name of the Hindu moon goddess [Hindi]
Devan	Variant of Devin; from the surname; fawn [Gaelic]; or the county Devon
Devin	From the surname; fawn [Gaelic]; or from the English county Devon
Devon	From the English county. Or from the surname; fawn [Gaelic]
Devyn	Variant of Devin; from the surname; fawn [Gaelic]; or from county of Devon
Dextra	Feminine form of Dexter; Or right-handed, skilled [Latin]
Dexy	Diminutive of Dextra; dyer [Old English]; or right-handed, skilled [Latin]
Dharma	Truth [Sanskrit]
Di	Diminutive of Dianna; divine [Indo-European]
Dia	Spanish form of Day; day
Diablo	Devil [Spanish/Latin]
Diabola	Devil [Latin]
Diamond	From the precious stone; invincible [Greek/Latin]
Diana	Variant of Dianna; divine [Indo-European]
Diane	Variant of Dianna; divine [Indo-European]
Dianna	Divine; heavenly [Indo-European]
Dianne	Variant of Dianna; divine [Indo-European]
Diantha	From the flower; heavenly flower [Greek]
Dillanne	Variant of Dillian; image of worship [Latin]
Dillian	Image of worship [Latin]
Dillon	Loyal [Irish]
Dina	Variant of Dinah; judge [Hebrew]
Dinah	Judge [Hebrew]
Dione	Variant of Dionne; goddess [Greek]
Dionisia	Feminine form of Dionysius; god from Nysa

Dionne	Feminine form of Dion; god/goddess [Greek]
Diva	Divine; goddess
Divina	Divine
Dixie	From the term for southern states of USA; ten [French]
Dodie	Diminutive of Dorothy; gift of God [Greek]
Dodo	Diminutive of Dorothy; gift of God [Greek]
Doe	Female deer
Dolcie	Variant of Dulcie; sweet [Latin]
Dollie	Diminutive of Dorothy; gift of God [Greek]
Dolly	Diminutive of Dorothy; gift of God [Greek]
Dolores	Sorrow [Spanish]
Domenica	Variant of Dominica; of the Lord [Latin]
Dominica	Of the Lord [Latin]
Dona	Variant of Donna; lady [Italian]
Donatella	Feminine diminutive of Donato; given by God [Italian]
Donna	Lady [Italian]
Dora	Diminutive of Dorothy, Isadora, Theodora etc
Dorcas	Gazelle [Greek]
Dorean	Variant of Doreen; Dora; diminutive of Dorothy, Isadora, Theodora etc.
Doreen	Variant of Doreen; Dora; diminutive of Dorothy, Isadora, Theodora etc
Doretta	Variant of Doreen; Dora; diminutive of Dorothy, Isadora, Theodora etc
Dorinda	Variant of Dora; diminutive of Dorothy, Isadora, Theodora etc.
Dorine	Variant of Doreen; Dora; diminutive of Dorothy, Isadora, Theodora etc.
Doris	Woman of Dorian tribe [Greek]
Dorita	Diminutive of Dora, Dorothy, Isadora, Theodora etc.
Dorothea	Variant of Dorothy; gift of God [Greek]
Dorothy	Gift of God [Greek]
Dory	Diminutive of Dorothy or Doris
Dot	Diminutive of Dorothy; gift of God [Greek]
Dottie	Diminutive of Dorothy; gift of God [Greek]
Douce	Sweet [French]
Dove	From the bird symbolizing peace
Drea	Diminutive of Andrea; strength [Greek]
Drina	Diminutive of Adriana; dark; from Adria
Dru	Diminutive of names beginning with Dru-
Drucilla	Strong [Latin]
Druella	Elf vision [Old German]
Duce	Variant of Douce; sweet [French]
Dulcie	Sweet [Latin]
Dusty	From nickname; dusty

E

Eabha	Irish form of Eve; breathe; live [Hebrew]
Eachna	Horse [Irish]
Eaden	Variant of Eden; from the Biblical garden; place of pleasure [Hebrew]
Ealanor	Variant of Eleanor; light, radiance [Arabic]
Earin	Variant of Erin; Ireland [Gealic]
Earline	Femine of Earl; from the aristocratic title earl
Earlene	Variant of Earline; feminine of Earl; from the aristocratic title
Early	Early
Earnestine	Variant of Ernestine; serious [German]
Eartha	From earth
East	East; the direction
Eastan	Variation of Easter; or from the Germanic spring goddess Eostre
Easter	From the Christian festival; from the Germanic spring goddess Eostre
Easton	Elaboration of East; or east town
Eba	Variant of Eva; breathe; live [Hebrew]
Ebele	Mercy; kindness [Igbo]
Ebony	From the tree and black wood [Egyptian]
Echo	Echo
Eddie	Diminutive of Edward. Edmund etc
Eden	From the Biblical garden; place of pleasure [Hebrew]
Edie	Diminutive of Edith; fortune of war [Old English]
Edina	Wealthy [Old Englsih]
Edith	Fortune of war; spoils of war [Old English]
Edlyn	Small, noble one [Old English]
Edna	English form of Eithne; grain, kernel [Irish]
Ednah	Variant of Edna; English form of Eithne; grain, kernel [Irish]
Edneisha	Elaborate form of Edna; English form of Eithne; grain, kernel [Irish]
Edvige	Variant of Edwige; French form of Hedwig; war [Old German]
Edvina	East European form of Edwina; rich friend [Old English]
Edwena	Variant of Edwina; rich friend [Old English]
Edwige	French form of Hedwig; war [Old German]
Edwina	Rich friend [Old English]
Effie	Diminutive of Euphemia; speaks good omens [Greek]
Eida	Variant of Ida; one who works [Old German]
Eidah	Variant of Ida; one who works [Old German]
Eileen	Desired. Or Irish variant of Helen; torch [Greek]
Eilidh	Gaelic for Eleanor; radiance [Arabic]. Scottish form of Helen; torch [Greek]

Elaine	Old French form of Helen; torch [Greek]
Elba	From the name of the Mediterranean island
Elbe	Variant of Elba; from the name of the island. Or from the name of the river
Elberta	High-born; shining [Old English]
Elbertha	Variant of Elberta; high-born; shining [Old English]
Eldora	Covered in gold [Spanish]
Eldorada	Elaborate form of Eldora; covered in gold [Spanish]
Elea	Diminutive of Eleanor; light [Arabic]. Variant of Helen; torch [Greek]
Eleanor	Light, radiance [Arabic]. Or variant of Helen; torch [Greek]
Eleanora	Variant of Eleanor; light, radiance [Arabic]. Variant of Helen; torch [Greek]
Eleanore	Variant of Eleanor; light, radiance [Arabic]. Variant of Helen; torch [Greek]
Elena	Variant of Helen; torch [Greek]
Elfreda	Elf strength [Old English]
Elfrida	Elf strength [Old English]
Elga	Sacred [Slavic]
Elgiva	Variant of Elga; sacred [Slavic]
Elia	Feminine diminutive of Elija; my God is Jehova [Hebrew]
Eliana	My God has answered [Hebrew]. Or from Roman name Aelius; sun [Greek]
Elisa	Diminutuve of Elisabeth/Elizabeth; oath of God [Hebrew]
Elisabeth	Variant of Elizabeth; oath of God [Hebrew]
Elise	Diminutive of Elisabeth/Elizabeth; oath of God [Hebrew]
Elisheba	Variant of Elisheva; oath of God [Hebrew]
Elisheva	Pledged to God [Hebrew]
Elissa	Diminutuve of Elisabeth/Elizabeth; oath of God [Hebrew]
Elixane	Basque variant of Elizabeth; oath of God [Hebrew]
Eliza	Dminutive of Elizabeth; oath of God [Hebrew]
Elizabeth	Oath of God [Hebrew]
Ella	Other [Norman French]. Or diminutive of Eleanor, Ellen etc.
Elle	Diminutive of Eleanor, Ellen etc. Or she [French]
Ellen	Variant of Helen; torch [Greek]
Elli	Diminutive of Eleanor, Ellen etc.
Ellie	Diminutive of Eleanor, Ellen etc.
Eloise	Healthy; wide [Old German/French]
Eloisia	Variant of Aloisia; famous in battle [Old German]
Elsa	Diminutive of Elisabeth/Elizabeth; oath of God [Hebrew]
Elsea	Variant of Elsie; diminutive of Elisabeth/Elizabeth; oath of God [Hebrew]
Elsie	Diminutive of Elisabeth/Elizabeth; oath of God [Hebrew]
Elspeth	Scottish form of Elisabeth/Elizabeth; oath of God [Hebrew]
Elvina	Variant of Alvina; elf friend [old English]
Elyse	Diminutive of Elisabeth/Elizabeth; oath of God [Hebrew]
Elysia	From Elysium, home of the blesses [Latin]
Em	Diminutive of Emily; rival [Latin]. Or of Emma; whole [Old German]
Ember	Emma + Amber. Or fire ember
Emelia	Variant of Amelia; industrious; striving [Old German]

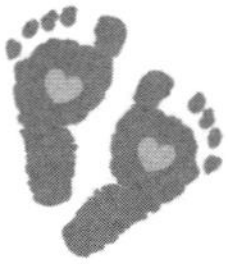

Emerald From the precious stone, reputed to impart love to the wearer [Greek]
Emerson From the surname; son of Emery
Emery From the surname; work; power [Old German]
Emilee Variant of Emily; rival [Latin]
Emilia Variant of Emily; rival [Latin]
Emily Rival [Latin]
Emira Feminine form of Amir; commander; prince [Arabic]
Emma Whole; universal [Old German]
Emmaline Variant of Emmeline; work [Old German]
Emmalyn Variant of Emmeline; work [Old German]. Or Emma + Lyn
Emmeline Work [Old German/Norman French]
Emmie Diminutive of Emily; rival [Latin]. Or of Emma; whole [Old German]
Emmy Diminutive of Emily; rival [Latin]. Or of Emma; whole [Old German]
Ena Diminutive of names containing -ena-
Enaya Variant of Inaya; concerned [Arabic]
Enfys Rainbow [Welsh]
England From the name of the country
Engracia Endowed with God's grace [Spanish/Latin]
Enid Soul; life [Welsh]
Enola Solitary [Native American]
Epiphany From the Christian festival; sudden perception [Old English]
Eppie Diminutive of Euphemia; speaks good omens [Greek]
Erendira She who smiles [Spanish]
Erga Yearning [Hebrew]
Erica Feminine form of Eric; always ruler [Old Norse]
Ericka Variant of Erica; always ruler [Old Norse]
Erika Variant of Erica; always ruler [Old Norse]
Erin Ireland [Gealic]
Erma Variant of Irma; whole; universal [Old German]
Ermintrude Universal strength [Old German]
Ernestine Serious [German]
Erykah Variant of Erica; always ruler [Old Norse]
Eryn Variant of Erin; Ireland [Gealic]
Erynne Variant of Erin; Ireland [Gealic]
Esma Variant of Esmé; loved; esteemed [old French]. Diminutive of Esmeralda; emerald
Esmaralda Variant of Esmeralda; emerald [Spanish; Portuguese]
Esme Variant of Esmé; loved; esteemed [old French]
Esmé Loved; esteemed [old French]
Esmée Feminine only variant of Esmé; loved; esteemed [old French]
Esmeralda Emerald [Spanish; Portuguese]
Essence Scent; intrinsic quality; spirit
Essie Diminutive of Estelle; star. Or of Esther
Esta Diminutive of Esther
Estella Variant of Estelle; star [Latin]

Estelle	Star [Latin]
Esther	Star [Persian]. Or from near-eastern goddess Ishtar
Ester	Variant of Esther; star [Persian]. Or from near-eastern goddess Ishtar
Estera	Bay [Spanish]
Ethel	Noble [Old English]
Ethelyn	Diminutive of Ethel; noble [Old English]
Etta	Home ruler [Old German]. Or of other names ending in etta
Ettie	Home ruler [Old German]. Or of other names ending in etta or ettie
Eugenia	Well born [Greek]
Eugenie	French variant of Eugenia; well born [Greek]
Eula	Diminutive of Eulalia; sweetly speaking [Greek]
Eulalia	Sweetly speaking [Greek]
Eunice	Good victory [Greek]
Euphemia	Speaks good omens [Greek]
Eustacia	Fruitful [Greek]
Eva	Latin form of Eve; breathe; live [Hebrew]
Evaline	Variant of Evelyn; desired [Old German]
Evalyn	Variant of Evelyn; desired [Old German]
Evangelina	Latin form of Evangeline; good news [Greek]
Evangeline	Good news [Greek]
Eve	Breathe; live [Hebrew]
Eveleen	Breathe; live [Hebrew]. Or variant of Evelyn; desired [Old German]
Evelina	Desired [Old German]. Or diminutive of Eve; breathe; live [Hebrew]
Eveline	Variant of Evelina/Evelyn; desired [Old German]
Evelyn	From the surname; desired [Old German]
Everly	From the surname; from the boar meadow [Old English]
Evette	Variant of Yvette; yew tree [Old German]
Evie	Breathe; live [Hebrew]. Or of Evelyn; desired [Old German]
Evonne	Variant of Yvonne; yew tree [Old German]
Evvie	Breathe; live [Hebrew]. Or of Evelyn; desired [Old German]

F

Fabia	Feminine form of Fabian; grower of beans [Latin]
Fabiana	Feminine form of Fabian; grower of beans [Latin]
Fabianne	Feminine form of Fabian; grower of beans [Latin]
Fabienne	Feminine form of Fabian; grower of beans [Latin]
Fae	Variant of Fay; fae; fairy [Old English]
Faina	Variant of Faine; joyful [Old English]. Or of Fawn; fawn
Faine	Joyful [Old English]

Fairuza Turquoise [Turkish]
Faith From the virtue, faith
Faithe Variant of Faith; from the virtue, faith
Fallon From the surname; leader [Irish Gaelic]
Fannie Diminutive of Frances; French/Frankish
Fanny Diminutive of Frances; French/Frankish
Fantasia Fantasy; imagination
Fantine Infant [French]
Fanya Russian & Slavic diminutive of Frances; French/Frankish
Fara Variant of Farah; happiness [Arabic]
Farah Happiness [Arabic]
Fargo From the name of the North Dakotan city
Farida Precious pearl [Arabic]
Fawn Young deer
Fay Fae; fairy [Old English]
Faydra Variant of Phaedra; bright [Greek]
Faye Variant of Fay; fae; fairy [Old English]
Fear Fear (perhaps of God)
Felicia Lucky, successful [Latin]
Felicity Happiness; good luck [English/Latin]
Fella Italian variant of Butterfly
Femie Diminutive of Euphemia; speaks good omens [Greek]
Fenella Anglicized form of Fionuala; white shouldered one [Gaelic]
Feodora Slavic form of Theodora; gift of God [Greek]
Ferdinanda A feminine form of Ferdinand; brave journey [Old German]
Ferdinande A feminine form of Ferdinand; brave journey [Old German]
Fern From the plant
Fernanda Feminine form of Ferdinand; brave journey [Old German]
Ferne Variant of Ferne; from the plant
Filomena Lover of song [Greek]
Fima Russian version of Seraphina; fiery ones; Biblical order of angels [Hebrew]
Finlay White warrior [Gaelic]
Finn Fair, white [Gaelic]
Fiona Fair [Gaelic]
Fionola Variant of Fionuala; white shouldered one [Gaelic]
Fionuala White shouldered one [Gaelic]
Flair Flair; talent
Flannery From the surname; red valour [Irish Gealic]
Flavia Golden; blonde [Latin]
Flaviana Elaborate form of Flavia; golden; blonde [Latin]
Fleur Flower [French]
Fleurette Diminutive of Fleur; flower [French]
Flick Diminutive of Felicity; happiness; good luck [English/Latin]
Flo Diminutive of Florence; flourishing; successful. Or of Flora; flower [Latin]

Flora	Flower [Latin]
Florence	Flourishing; successful [Latin]
Floretta	Diminutive of Flora; flower [Latin]
Florrie	Diminutive of Florence; flourishing; successful. Or of Flora; flower [Latin]
Flossie	Diminutive of Florence; flourishing; successful [Latin]
Flower	Flower
Fran	Diminutive of Frances etc; French/Frankish woman
Francene	Diminutive of Francoise/Frances; French/Frankish woman
Frances	Feminine form of Francis; French/Frankish woman
Francesca	Italian form of Frances; French/Frankish woman
Francine	Diminutive of Francoise/Frances; French/Frankish woman
Frankie	Diminutive of Frances etc; French/Frankish woman
Frannie	Diminutive of Frances etc; French/Frankish woman
Franny	Diminutive of Frances etc; French/Frankish woman
Freda	Diminutive of Winifred and other names ending in fred or freda
Freddie	Diminutive of Frederica, Freda and other named ending in fred or freda
Frederica	Feminine form of Frederick; peaceful ruler [Old German]
Freida	Variant of Frida; peace [Old German/Norse]
Freja	Danish form of Freya; lady [Old Norse]
Freya	Lady [OldNorse]
Frieda	Variant of Frida; peace [Old German/Norse]
Fritzie	Feminine form of Frederick; peaceful ruler [Old German]
Frona	Diminutive of Sophronia; sensible [Greek]

G

Gabby	Diminutive of Gabriel/Gabriella; God is my strength [Hebrew]
Gabriella	God is my strength [Hebrew]
Gabrielle	French form of Gabriella; God is my strength [Hebrew]
Gabrilla	Variant of Gabriella; God is my strength [Hebrew]
Gael	Variant of Gail; diminutive of Abigail; father's joy [Hebrew]
Gaetana	From Gaetana, Italy
Gaia	Earth mother [Greek]
Gail	Diminutive of Abigail; father's joy [Hebrew]
Gala	Diminutive of Galina; calm healer [Greek]
Gale	Variant of Gail; diminutive of Abigail; father's joy [Hebrew]
Galina	Femine form of Galen; calm healer [Greek]
Ganya	Clever [Hebrew]
Garbo	From an Italian nickname; polite; kind

Garda	Variant of Gerda; stronghold; enclosure [Norse]
Gardenia	From the flower
Garnet	From the precious stone; dark red [Old English].
Garnett	Variant of Garnet; from the precious stone; dark red [Old English]
Garnette	Variant of Garnet; from the precious stone; dark red [Old English]
Gavriela	Hebrew form of Gabriella; God is my strength {Hebrew]
Gayla	Variant of Gail; diminutive of Abigail; father's joy [Hebrew]
Gayle	Variant of Gail; diminutive of Abigail; father's joy [Hebrew]
Gaynor	Old form of Guinevere; fair phantom [Welsh]
Gemma	From nickname meaning precious stone [Italian]
Gena	Variant of Gina; diminutuve of Georgina, Regina etc.
Generosity	The virtue, generosity
Generva	Variant of Guinevere; fair phantom [Welsh]
Genessa	Variant of Genesis; birth; beginning [Greek]
Genesis	Birth; beginning [Greek]
Genette	Variant of Jeanette; God is gracious [Hebrew]
Geneva	Form of Genevieve; kinswoman [Germanic/Celtic]. Or from the Swiss city
Geneviève	Kinswoman [Germanic/Celtic]
Genevieve	English form of Geneviève; kinswoman [Germanic/Celtic]
Genie	Diminutive of Eugenia; well born [Greek]
Georgeanna	Variant of Georgiana; farmer [Old German]
Georgene	Variant of Georgina; farmer [Old German]
Georgia	Feminine form of George; farmer [Old German]. Or from the US state
Georgiana	Feminine form of George; farmer [Old German]
Georgie	Diminutive of Georgia, Georgina, Georgiana etc
Georgina	Feminine form of George; farmer [Old German]
Geraldine	Femine form of Gerald; rule of the spear [Old German]
Gerda	Stronghold; enclosure [Norse
Gerry	Diminutive of Geraldine; rule of the spear [Old German]
Gertie	Diminutive of Gertrude; strong spear [Old German]
Gertrude	Strong spear [Old German]
Gervasia	Feminine form of Gervaise; servant spear [Old German]
Gesine	Strength of a spear [Old German]
Ghislaine	Pledge [Old German]
Gianna	Diminutive of Giovanna or Joanna; God is gracious [Hebrew]
Gilda	Covered with gold
Gill	Diminutive of Gillian; downey-bearded [Greek]
Gillian	Feminine form of Julian; downey-bearded [Greek]
Gina	Diminutive of names ending in -gina or -ginia, e.g. Georgina, Virginia
Ginger	From the reddish spice. Or diminutive of Virginia; maid, virgin [Latin]
Ginnie	Diminutive of Virginia; maid, virgin [Latin]
Ginny	Diminutive of Virginia; maid, virgin [Latin]
Gisella	Variant of Giselle; hostage; pledge [Old German]
Giselle	Hostage; pledge [old German]

Giacinta Italian for hyacinth [Greek]
Giacintha Variant of Giacintha; hyacinth [Greek]
Gilenia Variant of Gillian; feminine form of Julian; downey-bearded [Greek]
Gita Good [Sanskrit]
Gladys Country [Welsh]. Or Welsh form of Claudia; lame
Glenda Pure and good [Welsh]
Glenna From the Scottish surname meaning of the glen/valley [Gaelic]
Glennishia Elaborate form of Glenna; of the glen/valley [Gaelic]
Glenys Pure; holy [Welsh]
Gloria Glory [Latin]
Gloriana Elaborate form of Gloria; glory [Latin]
Glynda Variant of Glenna; of the glen/valley [Gaelic]
Goldie From a nickname for blonde woman; gold colour
Grace The virtue, grace [Latin]
Gracelyn Made from Grace + Lyn
Gracia Spanish variant of Grace; the virtue, grace
Gracie Diminutive of Grace; the virtue, grace
Gray From the English surname; grey
Greer From a Scottish surname related to Gregor; watchful
Greta Diminutive of Margareta; pearl [Greek/Sanskrit]
Gretchen Diminutive of Margareta; pearl [Greek/Sanskrit]
Gretel Diminutive of Greta/Margaret; pearl [Greek/Sanskrit]
Gretna Variant of Greta; pearl [Greek]; Or from Gretna, Scotland
Grisel Variant of Griselda; grey battle [old German]
Griselda Grey battle [old German]
Grizel Variant of Griselda; grey battle [old German]
Guinevere Fair phantom [Welsh]
Gunhilda Battle maiden [Old Norse]
Gunna Diminutive of Gunhilda; battle maiden [Old Norse]
Gussie Diminutive of Augusta; great [Latin]
Gwen Fair; blessed [Welsh]. Or diminutive of Gwendolyn [fair browed; white ring]
Gwenda Fair and good [Welsh]
Gwendolen Variant of Gwendolyn; fair browed; white ring [Welsh]
Gwendoline Variant of Gendolyn; fair browed; white ring [Welsh]
Gwendolyn Fair browed; white ring [Welsh]
Gwenevere Variant of Guinivere; fair phantom [Welsh]
Gwyneth Fair; blessed [Welsh]
Gypsy Gypsy; wanderer

H

Habiba Beloved; sweetheart [North African]
Hacintha Variant of Jacinta; hyacinth {Greek]
Hadar Ornament; respect; glory [Hebrew]
Hadara Variant of Hadar; ornament; respect; glory [Hebrew]
Haddie Variant of Hattie; diminutive of Harriet; home ruler [Old German]
Hadiya Guide to righteousness [Arabic]
Hadley From an English surname; of the heather field
Hadria Variant of Adriana; dark; from Adria [Latin, Italian]
Hadrienne Variant of Adriana; dark; from Adria [Latin, Italian]
Hafsa Gathering [Arabic]
Hagar forsaken; flight [Hebrew]
Hailee Variant of Hayley; from the surname; of the hay clearing [Old English]
Hailey Variant of Hayley; from the surname; of the hay clearing [Old English]
Haley Variant of Hayley; from the surname; of the hay clearing [Old English]
Halima Gentle; compassionate [African]
Halle From the surname Hall; one who lives or works in a hall/manor house
Hallie Diminutive of Harriet; home ruler [Old German]
Hanako Flower child [Japanese]
Hanifa True believer [Arabic]
Hannah Grace; favour [Hebrew]
Happy Happy, cheerful in nature
Harley From the surname; hare woodland [Old English]
Harlow From the surname; of the rock hill; of the army hill [Old English]
Harmonie Variant of Harmony
Harmony Harmony
Harper From the surname; one who plays or makes harps
Harriet English for Henriette; feminine of Harry/Henry; home ruler [Old German]
Harriett Variant of Harriet; home ruler [Old German]
Harriette Variant of Harriet; home ruler [Old German]
Hattie Diminutive of Harriet; home ruler [Old German]
Hatty Diminutive of Harriet; home ruler [Old German]
Haven Haven; safe place
Hayden From the surname; of the hay hill/hay valley
Haylee Variant of Hayley; from the surname; of the hay clearing [Old English]
Hayleigh Variant of Hayley; from the surname; of the hay clearing [Old English]
Hayley From the surname; of the hay clearing [Old English]
Haylie Variant of Hayley; from the surname; of the hay clearing [Old English]

Haze	Diminutive of Hazel; hazel tree, or the nut colour
Hazel	Hazel tree, or the nut colour
Heather	From the shrub
Heaven	Heaven, paradise
Hedwig	War [German]
Heidi	Diminutive of Adelheid; noble and kind [Old German]
Helen	Torch [Greek]
Helena	Variant of Helen; torch[Greek]
Helenka	Polish diminutive of Helen; torch [Greek]
Helga	Successful; prosperous [Norse]
Hellen	Variant of Helen; torch [Greek]
Henley	From the surname; from name of the town; high meadow
Henrietta	Feminine form of Henry; home ruler [Old German]
Henriette	Variant of Henrietta; feminine form of Henry; home ruler [Old German]
Hereswith	Strength of the army [Old English]
Hermia	Feminine form of Hermes; messenger [Greek]
Hermione	Feminine derivation of Hermes; messenger; stone; cairn [Greek]
Hester	Latin form of Esther; star [Persian]. Or from near-eastern goddess Ishtar
Hetty	Diminutive of Henrietta; home ruler [Old German]. Star [Persian]
Hilary	Cheerful [Latin/Greek]
Hilda	Battle [Old German]
Hildegarde	Comrade in battle [Old German]
Hildred	Battle counsellor [Old German]
Hillary	Variant of Hilary; cheerful [Latin/Greek]
Hollie	Variant of Holly; from the holly tree
Hollis	From the surname; living near the holly trees [Old English]
Holly	From the holly tree
Honesty	Honesty
Honey	Honey
Honor	Variant of Honour; the vrtue
Honora	Variant of Honour; the virtue
Honoria	Variant of Honour; the virtue
Honour	The virtue, honour
Hope	The virtue, hope
Horatia	Feminine form of Horatio/Horrace; of the time/season/hour [Greek]
Hortense	Of the garden [Latin]
Hosanna	Deliver us [Hebrew]
Hosefina	Spanish form of Josephine, feminine form of Joseph; he will add [Hebrew]
Hoshi	Star [Japanese]
Hunter	Hunter
Hurricane	Hurricane [Native American]
Hyacinth	From the flower
Hylda	Variant of Hilda; battle [Old German]

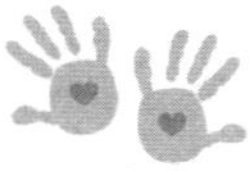

I

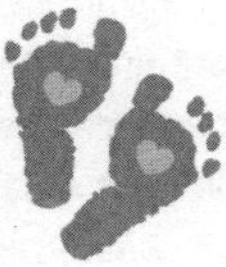

Iantha Variant of Iantha; purple flower [Greek]
Ianthe Purple flower [Greek]
Ibane Basque form of Yvonne; feminine diminutive of Yves/Ivo; yew tree
Iberia From the name of the Spanish & Portuguese peninsula
Ibbie Diminutive of Isabel; western form of Elizabeth; oath of God
Ida One who works [Old German]
Idella Elaborate form of Ida; one who works [Old German]
Ignacia Feminine form of Ignatius; from a Roman family name; fire; burning; ardent
Ignatia Feminine form of Ignatius; from a Roman family name; fire; burning; ardent
Ilaria Italian form of Hilary; cheerful [Latin/Greek]
Ilene Variant of Eileen; desired [Gaelic]
Ilona Joy, happiness [Finnish]. Or Hungarian variant of Helen; light [Greek]
Imagine Imagine
Imala Strong-minded [Native American]
Imani Faith [Arabic]
Imara Firm [Kiswahili]
Imelda Universal fight [Old German]
Imogen Maiden [Gaelic]
Imogene Variant of Imogen; maiden [Gaelic]
Ina Diminutive of names ending in -ina
Inaya Concerned [Arabic]
India From the country
Indiana From the US state; land of the Indians
Indigo From the colour
Inez Engish form of Inés, the Spanish form of Agnes; pure one [Greek]
Inga Gaurded by Ing [Old Norse]
Inka Polish form of Philippa; friend of horses
Ino Mythological Queen of Thebes [Greek]; wild boar [Japanese]
Iola Variant of Iole; violet [Greek]
Iole Violet [Greek]
Iona From the Scottish island; island [Old Norse]
Ione Violet flower [Greek]
Ireland From the country
Irena Variant of Irene; peace [Greek]
Irene Peace [Greek]
Iris Rainbow; iris flower; part of the eye [Greek]
Irma Variant of Emma; whole; universal [Old German]
Isa Strong-willed [German]. Or diminutive of names beginning with Isa-

Isabel Western form of Elizabeth; oath of God [Hebrew]
Isabella Latin form of Isabel; western form of Elizabeth; oath of God [Hebrew]
Isabelle French form of Isabel; western form of Elizabeth; oath of God [Hebrew]
Isadora Variant of Isidora; gift of Isis [Greek]
Isbel Variant of Isabel; western form of Elizabeth; oath of God [Hebrew]
Ishbel Scottish variant of Isabel; western form of Elizabeth; oath of God [Hebrew]
Isidora Gift of Isis [Greek]
Isla Variant of Islay; from the Scottish island
Islay From the Scottish island
Ismay Variant of Esme; beloved; esteemed [Old French]
Isolde Ice ruler [Welsh]
Isotta Italian form of Isolde; ice ruler [Welsh]
Issy Diminutive of Isabel and other names beginning with -is
Ivonnette Diminutive of Yvonne; yew tree [Old German], Or knowing [Celtic]
Ivory Ivory; white, pale
Ivy From the plant
Izabelle Variant of Isabel; western form of Elizabeth; oath of God [Hebrew]
Izzy Diminutive of Isabel and other names beginning with -is/-iz

J

Jaci Diminutive of Jacqueline; supplanter; or may God protect [Hebrew]
Jacinta Spanish form of Hyacinth
Jacki Diminutive of Jacqueline; supplanter; or may God protect [Hebrew]
Jackie Diminutive of Jacqueline; supplanter; or may God protect [Hebrew]
Jacklyn Variant of Jacqueline; supplanter; or may God protect [Hebrew]
Jaclyn Variant of Jacqueline; supplanter; or may God protect [Hebrew]
Jacqueline Feminine of Jacques; holder of the heel, or may God protect [Hebrew]
Jacquetta Feminine diminutive of Jacques; supplanter; or may God protect [Hebrew]
Jacqui Diminutive of Jacqueline; supplanter; or may God protect [Hebrew]
Jada Elaborate form of Jade; from the precious stone
Jade From the precious stone
Jaden God has heard; judge; thankful [Hebrew]
Jadyn Variant of Jaden; God has heard; judge; thankful [Hebrew]
Jaida Variant of Jada; elaborate form of Jade; from the precious stone
Jaiden Variant of Jaden; God has heard; judge; thankful [Hebrew]
Jaime Variant of Jamie; Scots diminutive of James; supplanter [Hebrew]
Jaimie Variant of Jamie; Scots diminutive of James; supplanter [Hebrew]
Jaki Diminutive of Jacqueline; supplanter; or may God protect [Hebrew]

Jami Variant of Jamie; Scots diminutive of James; supplanter [Hebrew]
Jamie Scots diminutive of James; supplanter [Hebrew]
Jan Diminutive of Janet, Janice and other names beginning with Jan-
Janae Elaborate form of Jane; feminine form of John; God is gracious [Hebrew]
Jancis Jan + Francis
Jane Feminine form of John; God is gracious [Hebrew]
Janeka Diminutive of Jane, feminine form of John; God is gracious [Hebrew]
Janel Diminutive of Jane, feminine form of John; God is gracious [Hebrew]
Janella Diminutive of Jane; feminine form of John; God is gracious [Hebrew]
Janelle Modern diminutive of Jane; feminine form of John; God is gracious [Hebrew]
Janene Diminutive of Jeanne, French feminine form of John; God is gracious [Hebrew]
Janessa Elaborate form of Jane, feminine form of John; God is gracious [Hebrew]
Janet Diminutive of Jane, feminine form of John; God is gracious [Hebrew]
Janetta Diminutive of Jane, a feminine form of John; God is gracious [Hebrew]
Janette Diminutve of Jane; feminine form of John; God is gracious [Hebrew]
Janey Diminutive of Jane, feminine form of John; God is gracious [Hebrew]
Janice Elaborate form of Jane, feminine form of John; God is gracious [Hebrew]
Janie Diminutive of Jane, feminine form of John; God is gracious [Hebrew]
Janine French feminine form of John; God is gracious [Hebrew]
Janis Variant of Janice, feminine form of John; God is gracious [Hebrew]
Janna Feminine form of Jan/John; God is gracious [Hebrew]. Diminutive of Janet
Jannah Feminine form of Jan/John; diminutive of Janet; God is gracious [Hebrew]
Jannette Diminutve of Jane; feminine form of John; God is gracious [Hebrew]
Jannine Diminutive of Jane, feminine form of John; God is gracious [Hebrew]
Jaqueline Variant of Jacqueline; supplanter; or may God protect [Hebrew]
Jaquelyn Variant of Jacqueline; supplanter; or may God protect [Hebrew]
Jasmin Variant of Jasmine; from the name of the plant [Persian]
Jasmine From the name of the plant [Persian]
Jasmyn Variant of Jasmine; from the name of the plant [Persian]
Jayda Variant of Jada; elaborate form of Jade; from the precious stone
Jayde Variant of Jade; from the precious stone
Jayden Variant of Jaden; God has heard; judge; thankful [Hebrew]
Jaye Feminine form of Jay; diminutive of names beginning with J-
Jayla Elaborate form of Jay; diminutive of names beginning with J-
Jaylee Jay + Lee
Jaylen Elaborate form of Jay; diminutive of names beginning with J-
Jaylene Elaborate form of Jay; diminutive of names beginning with J-
Jaylin Elaborate form of Jay; diminutive of names beginning with J-
Jaylyn Elaborate from of Jay; diminutive of names beginning with J-
Jayma Variant of Jamie; Scots diminutive of James; supplanter [Hebrew]
Jayme Variant of Jamie; Scots diminutive of James; supplanter [Hebrew]
Jayna Variant of Jane, feminine form of John; God is gracious [Hebrew]
Jayne Variant of Jane, feminine form of John; God is gracious [Hebrew]
Jaynie Diminutive of Jayne, feminine form of John; God is gracious [Hebrew]

Jazlyn	Unknown meaning; possibly Jasmine + Lyn
Jazmin	Variant of Jasmine; from the plant [Persian]
Jazmine	Variant of Jasmine; from the plant [Persian]
Jazmyn	Variant of Jasmine; from the plant [Persian]
Jean	Variant of Jane; feminine form of John; God is gracious [Hebrew]
Jeana	Variant of Jean, feminine form of John; God is gracious [Hebrew]
Jeane	Variant of Jean, feminine form of John; God is gracious [Hebrew]
Jeanette	Variant of Jeannette, French dimuntive of Jeanne; God is gracious [Hebrew]
Jeanie	Diminutive of Jean, feminine form of John; God is gracious [Hebrew]
Jeanine	Diminutive of Jean. Feminine form of John; God is gracious [Hebrew]
Jeanna	Variant of Jean, feminine form of John; God is gracious [Hebrew]
Jeanne	French form of Jane/Jean; God is gracious [Hebrew]
Jeannette	French diminutive of Jeanne; God is gracious [Hebrew]
Jeannie	Diminutive of Jean. Feminine forms of John; God is gracious [Hebrew]
Jeannine	Diminutive of Jean. Feminine forms of John; God is gracious [Hebrew]
Jemima	Dove [Hebrew]
Jemma	Variant of Gemma; from Italian nickname meaning gem
Jen	Diminutive of Jennifer, Cornish variant of Guinivere; white phantom [Welsh]
Jena	Diminutive of Jennifer, Cornish variant of Guinivere; white phantom [Welsh]
Jenae	Diminutive of Jennifer, Cornish variant of Guinivere; white phantom [Welsh]
Jenelle	Jen + -elle
Jenessa	Jen + -essa
Jeni	Diminutive of Jennifer, Cornish variant of Guinivere; white phantom [Welsh]
Jenifer	Varaint of Jennifer, a Cornish variant of Guinivere; white phantom [Welsh]
Jenn	Diminutive of Jennifer, Cornish variant of Guinivere; white phantom [Welsh]
Jenna	Diminutive of Jennifer; white phantom [Welsh]; God is gracious [Hebrew]
Jenni	Diminutive of Jennifer; white phantom [Welsh]; God is gracious [Hebrew]
Jennica	Jennifer + Jessica
Jennie	Diminutive of Jennifer; white phantom [Welsh]; God is gracious [Hebrew]
Jennifer	Cornish variant of Guinivere; white phantom [Welsh]
Jenny	Diminutive of Jennifer; white phantom [Welsh]; God is gracious [Hebrew]
Jeri	Diminutive of Geraldine, feminine of Gerald; rule of the spear [Old German]
Jerri	Diminutive of Geraldine, feminine of Gerald; rule of the spear [Old German]
Jerrie	Diminutive of Geraldine, feminine of Gerald; rule of the spear [Old German]
Jerry	Diminutive of Geraldine, feminine of Gerald; rule of the spear [Old German]
Jess	Diminutive of Jessica; to behold [Hebrew]
Jessa	Diminutive of Jessica; to behold [Hebrew]
Jessalyn	Jessa + -lyn
Jessamine	Variant of Jasmine; from the plant [Persian]
Jessamy	Variant of Jasmine; from the plant [Persian]
Jessamyn	Variant of Jasmine; from the plant [Persian]
Jessi	Diminutive of Jessica; to behold [Hebrew]
Jessica	To behold [Hebrew]
Jessie	Diminutive of Jessica; to behold [Hebrew]. God is gracious [Hebrew]

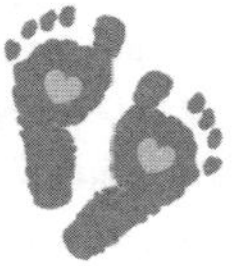

Jessika	Variant of Jessica; to behold [Hebrew]
Jessye	Diminutive of Jessica; to behold [Hebrew]
Jewel	Precious stone. Or from the surname; generous prince [Old Breton]
Jezebel	Not exalted [Hebrew]
Jill	Diminutive of Gillian; feminine form of Julian; downey-bearded [Greek]
Jillian	Variant of Gillian; feminine form of Julian; downey-bearded [Greek]
Jillie	Diminutive of Gillian; feminine form of Julian; downey-bearded [Greek]
Jilly	Diminutive of Gillian; feminine form of Julian; downey-bearded [Greek]
Jimmy	Feminine form of James; supplanter [Hebrew]
Jinny	Diminutive of Virginia; virgin, maid [Latin]
Jo	Diminutive of Joan, Joanna, Josephine
Joan	Feminine form of John; God is gracious [Hebrew]
Joanie	Diminutive of Joan; feminine form of John; God is gracious [Hebrew]
Joann	Variant of Joan, feminine form of John; God is gracious [Hebrew]
Joanna	Feminine form of John; God is gracious [Hebrew]
Joanne	Variant of Joanna, feminine form of John; God is gracious [Hebrew]
Jobeth	Jo + Beth
Jocasta	Shining moon [Greek]
Jocelin	Variant of Jocelyn; from Gaul [Old German]
Jocelyn	From Gaul [Old German]
Jodene	Woman from Judea [Hebrew]. Or feminine of Joseph; he will add [Hebrew]
Jodi	Woman from Judea [Hebrew]. Or feminine of Joseph; he will add [Hebrew]
Jodie	Variant of Jodi. Or a feminine form of Joseph; he will add [Hebrew]
Jody	Variant of Jodi. Or a feminine form of Joseph; he will add [Hebrew]
Joella	Feminine form of Joel; Jehova is God [Hebrew]
Joelle	Feminine form of Joel; Jehova is God [Hebrew]
Joetta	Elaborate form of Jo
Joey	Diminutive of Joanna or Joseohine
Johanna	Variant of Joanna, feminine form of John; God is gracious [Hebrew]
Johna	Feminine form of John; God is gracious [Hebrew]
Johnie	Feminine diminutive of John; God is gracious [Hebrew]
Johnna	Feminine form of John; God is gracious [Hebrew]
Johnnie	Feminine diminutive of John; God is gracious [Hebrew]
Joi	Variant of Joy; joy
Jojo	Diminutive of names beginning with Jo-
Joleen	Variant of Jolene; Jo + -lene
Jolene	Jo + -lene
Jolie	Pretty [French]
Jonelle	Feminine form of John; God is gracious [Hebrew]
Jonette	Feminine form of John; God is gracious [Hebrew]
Joni	Diminutive of Joan; feminine form of John; God is gracious [Hebrew]
Jonie	Diminutive of Joan; feminine form of John; God is gracious [Hebrew]
Jonquil	From the flower
Jools	Diminutive of Julia/Julie; feminine form of Julius; downy-bearded [Greek]

Jordan	From the name of the river
Jordana	Variant of Jordan; from the name of the river
Jordyn	Variant of Jordan; from the name of the river
Jorie	Diminutive of Marjorie, medieval form of Margaret; pearl [Greek]
Jorja	Modern variant of Georgia; feminine form of George; farmer [Old German].
Joselyn	Variant of Jocelyn; from Gaul [Old German]
Josepha	Feminine form of Joseph; he will add [Hebrew]
Josephina	Variant of Josephine, feminine form of Joseph; he will add [Hebrew]
Josephine	Feminine form of Joseph; he will add [Hebrew]
Josie	Diminutive of Josephine, feminine form of Joseph; he will add [Hebrew]
Joslyn	Variant of Jocelyn; from Gaul [Old German]
Joss	Diminutive of Jocelyn; from Gaul [old German]
Josslyn	Variant of Jocelyn; from Gaul [Old German]
Joy	Joy
Joyce	Lord [Old Breton]; influenced by joise, rejoice [Old English]
Joye	Variant of Joy
Jude	Diminutive of Judith; woman of Judea [Hebrew]
Judie	Diminutive of Judith; woman of Judea [Hebrew]
Judith	Woman of Judea [Hebrew]
Judy	Diminutive of Judith; woman of Judea [Hebrew]
Jules	Diminutive of Julia/Julie; feminine form of Julius; downy-bearded [Greek]
Julia	Feminine form of Julius; downy-bearded [Greek]
Juliana	Feminine form of Julius; downy-bearded [Greek]
Julianna	Feminine form of Julius; downy-bearded [Greek]
Julie	French form of Julia; downy-bearded [Greek]
Juliet	Diminutive of Julia/Julie; feminine form of Julius; downy-bearded [Greek]
Juliette	Diminutive of Julia/Julie; feminine form of Julius; downy-bearded [Greek]
July	From the month named for Julius Caesar
June	From the month named for goddess Juno
Junia	Elaborate form of June; from the month named for the goddess Juno
Juniper	From the juniper tree/berry
Justice	From the surname; judge. Or justice
Justina	Feminine form of Justin; just [Latin]
Justine	Feminine form of Justin; just [Latin]
Justy	Diminutive of Justina/Justine; just [Latin]

K

Kacey	Variant of Casey; from the surname; vigilant [Irish]
Kacie	Variant of Casey; from the surname; vigilant [Irish]

Kae	Variant of Kay; diminutive of Katherine and other names beginning with K
Kaelea	Variant of Kaylee; Kay + -lee
Kaelee	Variant of Kaylee; Kay + -lee
Kaelyn	Variant of Kaylin; Kay + -lin
Kailee	Variant of Kaylee; Kay + -lee
Kailey	Variant of Kaylee; Kay + -lee
Kailyn	Variant of Kaylin; Kay + -lin
Kaitlin	Variant of Caitlin; Irish form of Kathleen/Katherine; pure [Greek]
Kaitlyn	Variant of Caitlin; Irish form of Kathleen/Katherine; pure [Greek]
Kaitlynn	Variant of Caitlin; Irish form of Kathleen/Katherine; pure [Greek]
Kaleigh	Variant of Kayleigh; ceilidh, social gathering [Gaelic]
Kaley	Variant of Kaylee; Kay + -lee
Kalie	Variant of Kaylee; Kay + -lee
Kalla	Variant of Calla; type of lily; beautiful [Greek]
Kallie	Variant of Callie; diminutive of Caroline; warrior [Old German]
Kalyn	Variant of Kaylin; Kay + -lin
Kamryn	Variant of Cameron; crooked nose [Gaelic]
Kandace	Variant of Candace; queen mother [Cushitic]
Kandi	Variant of Candy; sweet. Diminutive of Candace; queen mother [Cushitic]
Kara	Variant of Cara; beloved [Italian}
Karen	Danish diminutive of Katherine; pure [Greek]
Karena	Elaboration of Karen, diminutive of Katherine; pure [Greek]
Karenza	Variant of Kerensa; love [Cornish]
Karin	Swedish diminutive of Katherine; pure [Greek]
Karina	Elaborate form of Karin; Swedish diminutive of Katherine; pure [Greek]
Karissa	Variant of Charissa; grace; kindness [Greek]
Karlee	Variant of Carly/Carla; warrior [Old German]
Karolyn	Variant of Caroline; warrior [Old German]
Karrie	Variant of Carrie, diminutive of Caroline; warrior [Old German]
Karyn	Variant of Karen; dimuntive of Katherine; pure [Greek]
Karyna	Variant of Carina; form of Cara; beloved [Italian]
Kassandra	Variant of Cassandra; excell; shine [Greek]
Kassia	Variant of Cassia; vain; empty [Latin]
Kassidy	Variant of Cassidy; from the surname; curly-haired [Irish]
Kassy	Diminutive of Kassandra/Cassandra; excell; shine [Greek]
Kat	Diminutive of Katherine/Kathleen; pure [Greek]
Kate	Diminutive of Katherine; pure [Greek]
Katelin	Variant of Caitlin; Irish form of Kathleen/Katherine; pure [Greek]
Katelyn	Variant of Caitlin; Irish form of Kathleen/Katherine; pure [Greek]
Katelynn	Variant of Caitlin; Irish form of Kathleen/Katherine; pure [Greek]
Katey	Diminutive of Katherine; pure [Greek]
Katharine	Variant of Katherine; pure [Greek]
Katheryn	Variant of Katherine; pure [Greek]
Kathi	Diminutive of Katherine; pure [Greek]

Kathie Diminutive of Katherine; pure [Greek]
Kathleen Variant of Caitlin; Irish form of Kathleen/Katherine; pure [Greek]
Kathlyn Variant of Caitlin; Irish form of Kathleen/Katherine; pure [Greek]
Kathryn Variant of Katherine; pure [Greek]
Kathy Diminutive of Katherine; pure [Greek]
Katie Diminutive of Katherine; pure [Greek]
Katlin Variant of Caitlin; Irish form of Kathleen/Katherine; pure [Greek]
Katrin Diminutive of Katherine; pure [Greek]
Katrina Variant of Catriona, Gaelic form of Katherine; pure [Greek]
Katriona Variant of Catriona, Gaelic form of Katherine; pure [Greek]
Katy Diminutive of Katherine; pure [Greek]
Kay Diminutive of Katherine; pure [Greek]. And other names beginning with K
Kaycee Variant of Casey; from the surname; vigilant [Irish]
Kaydence Variant of Cadence; rhythm; inflection
Kaye Variant of Kay; diminutive of Katherine and other names beginning with K
Kayla Kay + -la
Kayleah Variant of Kaylee; Kay + -lee
Kaylee Kay + -lee
Kayleen Kay + leen
Kayleigh Variant of Kaylee; Kay + -lee. Or from ceilidh; social gathering [Gaelic]
Kayley Variant of Kaylee; Kay + -lee
Kaylie Variant of Kaylee; Kay + -lee
Kaylin Kay + -lin
Kayly Variant of Kaylee; Kay + -lee
Kaylyn Kay + -lyn
Kaylynn Variant of Kaylyn
Keanna Ke + Anna; favour; grace [Hebrew]
Keara Variant of Ciara, variant of Sierra; mountain range [Spanish]. Or black [Irish]
Keeleigh Variant of Keely; from the surname; slender [Irish]
Keeley Variant of Keely; from the surname; slender [Irish]
Keely From the surname; slender [Irish]
Keila Variant of Kayla; Kay + -la
Keira Variant of Kira/Ciara; black [Irish]
Kelcey Variant of Kelsey; from the surname; from Cenel's island [Old English]
Kelley Variant of Kelly; from the surname; bright-headed; war; church [Irish]
Kelly From the surname; bright-headed; war; church [Irish]
Kelsey From the surname; Cenel's island [Old English]
Kendal From the surname; from the valley of the River Kent
Kendall From the surname; from the valley of the River Kent
Kendra Feminine form of Ken/Kenneth; handsome; born of fire [Gaelic].
Kennedy From the surname; armoured head [Gaelic]
Kenya From the African country
Kenzie Contraction of MacKenzie; handsome [Gaelic]
Kerena Variant of Karena; elaborate form of Karen; pure

Keri	Variant of Kerry; from the Irish county; black [Irish]
Kerri	Variant of Kerry; from the Irish county; black [Irish]
Kerrie	Variant of Kerry; from the Irish county; black [Irish]
Kerry	From the Irish county; black [Irish]
Keziah	Cinnamon tree [Hebrew]
Khloe	Variant of Chloe; green shoot [Greek]
Kiara	Variant of Ciara; black [Irish]. Or variant of Sierra; mountain range [Spanish]
Kiarra	Variant of Ciara; black [Irish]. Or variant of Sierra; mountain range [Spanish]
Kierra	Variant of Ciara; black [Irish]. Or variant of Sierra; mountain range [Spanish]
Kiersten	Variant of Kirsten; Scandinavian form of Christine; Christian
Kiki	Diminutive of names containing the letter k
Kim	Diminutive of Kimberley. Or of Kimball; war chief; bold
Kimberlee	Variant of Kimberley; from the South African city
Kimberley	From the South African city
Kimberly	Variant of Kimberley; from the South African city
Kimmie	Diminutive of Kimberley or Kim
Kimmy	Diminutive of Kimberley or Kim
Kinley	From the surname; fair warrior [Gaelic]
Kinsley	From the surname; royal victory [Old English]
Kira	Variant of Ciara; black [Irish]. Or variant of Sierra; mountain range [Spanish]
Kirsten	Scandinavian form of Christine; Christian
Kirsty	Diminutive of Kirsten, Scandinavian form of Christine; Christian
Kit	Diminutive of Katherine; pure [Greek]
Kitty	Diminutive of Katherine; pure [Greek]
Kizzy	Diminutive of Keziah; cinnamon tree [Hebrew]
Kori	Variant of Corey; hollow-dweeler; spear [Old Norse]
Korrine	Variant of Corinne; maiden [Greek]
Kortney	Variant of Courtney; from the surname; short-nose [Norman French]
Kourtney	Variant of Courtney; from the surname; short-nose [Norman French]
Kris	Diminutive of Christine etc.; Christian
Krista	Diminutive of Kristina, variant of Christine; Christian
Kristal	Variant of Crystal; cut glass; ice [Greek]
Kristen	Variant of Krsitin, Scandinavian form of Christine; Christian
Kristi	Diminutive of Kristina/Christine; Christian
Kristina	Variant of Christine/Christina; Christian
Kristine	Variant of Christine/Christina; Christian
Kristy	Diminutive of Kristina/Christine; Christian
Krystal	Variant of Crystal; cut glass; ice [Greek]
Krystelle	Variant of Crystal; cut glass; ice [Greek]
Krysten	Variant of Krsitin, Scandinavian form of Christine; Christian
Krystina	Variant of Kristina/Christina; Christian
Krystle	Variant of Crystal; cut glass; ice [Greek]
Kyla	Feminine form of Kyle; from the Scottish surname meaning channel; strait
Kylee	Variant of Kylie; boomerang [Australian Aboriginal]. Feminine form of Kyle

Kyleigh Variant of Kylie; boomerang [Australian Aboriginal]. Feminine form of Kyle
Kylie Boomerang [Australian Aboriginal]. Feminine for Kyle; Scottish surname
Kym Variant of Kim. Or diminutive of Kimberley, from the South African city
Kyra Variant of Kira/Ciara; black [Irish]
Kyrie Throne [Persian]; lord [Greek]
Kyrsten Variant of Kirsten; Scandinavian form of Christine; Christian

L

Lacey Variant of Lacy; from the surname; from the town of Lassy, Normandy
Laci Variant of Lacy; from the surname; from the town of Lassy, Normandy
Lacy From the surname; from the town of Lassy, Normandy
Laila Variant of Layla; night [Arabic]
Lainey Variant of Laney, diminutive of Elaine; old French form of Helen; torch [Greek]
Lalia Diminutive of Eulalia; sweetly speaking [Greek]
Lana Beautiful child; little rock [Gaelic]. Or of Svetlana; light world [Slavic/Russian
Laney Diminutive of Elaine; old French form of Helen; torch [Greek]
Lara Diminutive of Larissa; citadel [Greek]
Laraine Variant of Lorraine; from the region of France
Larissa Citadel [Greek]
Lark From the songbird
Latisha Variant of Letitia; happiness [Latin]
Laura Feminine form of Laurus; laurel [Latin]
Laureen Diminutive of Laura; laurel [Latin]
Laurel From the laurel tree [Latin]
Lauren Feminine form of Laurence; from Laurentum in Ancient Rome [Latin]
Laurena Elaborate form of Lauren; from Laurentum in Ancient Rome [Latin]
Laurene Diminutive of Laura; laurel [Latin]
Laurie Diminutive of Laura; laurel [Latin]
Laurinda Variant of Lorinda; elaborate form of Laura
Lauryn Variant of Lauren; from Laurentum in Ancient Rome [Latin]
Lavender From the flower
Lavern Variant of Laverne; from the place of alder trees [French]
Laverne From the place of alder trees [French]
Lavina Variant of Lavinia; unknown meaning [Etruscan]
Lavinia Lavinia was the wife of Aeneas who named city of Lavinium after her
Lavonne La- + Yvonne; yew tree [Old German]. Or knowing [Celtic]
Layla Night [Arabic]

Leah	Weary [Hebrew]
Leann	Lee + Ann; grace [Hebrew]
Leanna	Variant of Lianna, diminutive of Julianna
Leanne	Lee + Anne; grace [Hebrew]
Leanora	Diminutive of Eleanora; light, radiance [Arabic]
Leatrice	Leah + Beatrice; weary traveller
Lee	From the surname; from a clearing [Old English]
Leeann	Lee + Ann
Leesa	Variant of Lisa; diminutive of Elizabeth; oath of God [Hebrew]
Leigh	From the surname, a variant of Lee; from a clearing [Old English]
Leila	Variant of Layla; night [Arabic]
Leilah	Variant of Layla; night [Arabic]
Lela	Variant of Layla; night [Arabic]
Lena	Diminutive of Helena, Magdalena, Yelena and other names endind in -lena
Lenora	Diminutive of Eleonora; light; radiance [Arabic]
Lenore	Diminutive of Eleanor; light; radiance [Arabic]
Leola	Feminine form of Leo; lion [Latin]
Leona	Fminine form of Leon; lion [Greek]
Leone	Variant of Leona; lion [Greek]
Leonie	Variant of Leona; lion [Greek]
Lesia	Diminutive of Alesia; variant of Alicia; noble one [Greek].
Lesley	Variant of Leslie; from a Scottish surname; garden of holly [Gaelic]
Leslie	From a Scottish surname; garden of holly [Gaelic]
Lesly	Variant of Leslie; from a Scottish surname; garden of holly [Gaelic]
Lessie	Diminutive of names containing “les”, e.g. Leslie
Leta	Glad [Latin]
Letha	Diminutive of Aletha; truth [Greek]
Letitia	Happiness [Latin]
Lettice	Variant of Letitia; happiness [Latin]
Lettie	Diminutive of Letitia/Lettice; happiness [Latin]
Letty	Diminutive of Letitia/Lettice; happiness [Latin]
Lexa	Diminutive of Alexa or Alexandra; the defender [Greek]
Lexi	Diminutive of Alexa or Alexandra; the defender [Greek]
Lexia	Diminutive of Alexa or Alexandra; the defender [Greek]
Lexie	Diminutive of Alexa or Alexandra; the defender [Greek]
Lexine	Diminutive of Alexa or Alexandra; the defender [Greek]
Lexus	Diminutive of Alexus; the defender [Greek]
Lexy	Diminutive of Alexa or Alexandra; the defender [Greek]
Leyla	Variant of Layla; night [Arabic]
Liana	Diminutive of names ending in -liana, e.g. Juliana
Lianne	Variant of Leanne; Lee + Anne; grace [Hebrew]
Libbie	Diminutive of Elizabeth or Isabel; oath of God [Hebrew]
Libby	Diminutive of Elizabeth or Isabel; oath of God [Hebrew]
Liberty	Liberty; freedom

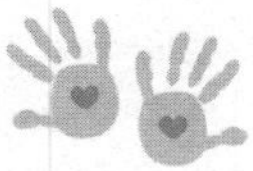

Liddy	Diminutive of Elizabeth; oath of God [Hebrew].
Lila	Variant of Layla; night [Arabic]
Lilac	From the name of the shrub [Arabic/Persian]
Lilian	Variant of Lillian; elaborate form of Lily; the flower. Diminutive of Elizabeth
Liliana	Elaborate form of Lillian/Lily/Elizabeth
Lilias	Scottish form of Lillian; elaborate form of Lily
Lillibet	Diminutive of Elizabeth; oath of God [Hebrew]
Lilibeth	Diminutive of Elizabeth; oath of God [Hebrew]
Lillia	Elaborate form of Lily. Or diminutive of Lillian
Lillian	Elaborate form of Lily; the flower. Or diminutive of Elizabeth; oath of God
Lilliana	Elaborate form of Lily/Lillian/Elizabeth
Lillie	Variant of Lily; the flower, symbolizing purity
Lilly	Variant of Lily; the flower, symbolizing purity
Lily	From the flower, symbolizing purity
Lina	Diminutive of names ending in -lina
Linda	Beautiful [Spanish/Portuguese]; tender, soft [Old German]
Lindsay	From the surname; from Lindsay, Lincolnshire
Lindsey	Variant of Lindsay; from the surname; from Lindsay, Lincolnshire
Lindy	Diminutive of Linda; beautiful [Spanish/Portuguese]; tender, soft [Old German]
Linette	Variant of Lynette; image/idol. Or diminutive of Lynn; of the lake [Welsh]
Linnaea	From the name of the flower
Linnet	Variant of Lynette; image/idol. Diminutive of Lynn; of the lake [Welsh]. From the bird
Linnette	Variant of Lynette; image/idol. Diminutive of Lynn; of the lake [Welsh]
Linnie	Diminutive of Linda; beautiful [Spanish/Portuguese]; tender, soft [Old German]
Linsay	Variant of Lindsay; from the surname; from Lindsay, Lincolnshire
Linzi	Variant of Lindsay; from the surname; from Lindsay, Lincolnshire
Lisa	Diminutive of Elizabeth/Elizabeth; oath of God [Hebrew]
Lise	Diminutive of Elizabeth/Elizabeth; oath of God [Hebrew]
Liselotte	Lise + Charlotte
Lisette	Diminutive of Elizabeth/Elizabeth; oath of God [Hebrew]
Lisha	Diminutive of names ending in -licia
Lissa	Diminutive of Melissa; bee [Greek]
Lita	Diminutive of names ending in -lita
Liv	Diminutive of Olivia; olive [Latin]. Feminine form of Oliver; elf warrior [Old German]
Livia	Diminutive of Olivia; olive [Latin]. Feminine form of Oliver; elf warrior [Old German]
Livvy	Diminutive of Olivia; olive [Latin]. Feminine form of Oliver; elf warrior [Old German]
Liz	Diminutive of Elizabeth; oath of God [Hebrew]
Liza	Diminutive of Elizabeth; oath of God [Hebrew]
Lizbeth	Diminutive of Elizabeth; oath of God [Hebrew]
Lizette	Diminutive of Elizabeth; oath of God [Hebrew]
Lizzie	Diminutive of Elizabeth; oath of God [Hebrew]
Lizzy	Diminutive of Elizabeth; oath of God [Hebrew]
Logan	From the Scottish surname; from the little hollow [Gaelic]
Lois	Desirable [Greek]

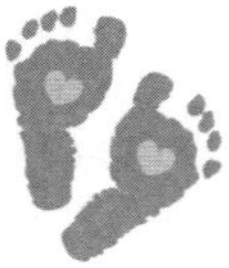

Lola	Diminutive of Dolores; sorrow [Spanish]
London	From the name of the city
Londyn	Variant of London; from the name of the city
Lora	Variant of Laura; laurel [Latin]. Or dimuntive of Eleonora; light; radiance [Arabic]
Loraine	Varriant of Lorraine; from the region of France
Lorayne	Variant of Lorraine; from the region of France
Loreen	Elaborate form of Lora. Dimuntive of Eleonora; light; radiance [Arabic]
Lorelei	Temptress; alluring [Old German]
Lorelle	Variant of Lauren; from Laurentum in Ancient Rome [Latin]
Loren	Variant of Lauren; from Laurentum in Ancient Rome [Latin]
Lorena	Variant of Lauren; from Laurentum in Ancient Rome [Latin]
Lorene	Elaborate form of Lora. Dimuntive of Eleonora; light; radiance [Arabic]
Loretta	Elaborate form of Lora. Dimuntive of Eleonora; light; radiance [Arabic].
Lori	Diminutive of Laura; laurel [Latin]. Or of Lorraine; from the region of France
Lorie	Diminutive of Laura; laurel [Latin]. Or of Lorraine; from the region of France
Lorinda	Elaborate form of Lora/Laura; laurel [Latin]
Lorna	Probably feminine form of Lorne; from Lorne in Scotland
Lorraine	From the region of France
Lorri	Diminutive of Laura; laurel [Latin]. Or of Lorraine; from the region of France
Lorrie	Diminutive of Laura; laurel [Latin]. Or of Lorraine; from the region of France
Lottie	Diminutive of Charlotte; feminine diminutive of Charles; warrior [Old German]
Lotus	From the name of the flower [Greek]
Lou	Diminutive of Louise; feminine form of Louis; famous in battle [Old German]
Louella	Lou + -ella
Louisa	Feminine form of Louis; famous in battle [Old German]
Louise	French feminine form of Louis; famous in battle [Old German]
Love	Love
Luana	Happy, contented [Hawaiian]
Luann	Variant of Luana; happy, contented [Hawaiian]. Or Lou + Ann
Luanna	Variant of Luana; happy, contented [Hawaiian]. Or Lou + Anna
Luanne	Variant of Luana; happy, contented [Hawaian]. Or Lou + Anne
Lucetta	Diminutive of Lucia; light [Latin]
Lucia	Feminine form of Lucius; light [Latin]
Lucile	Variant of Lucille; light [Latin]
Lucille	Light [Latin]
Lucinda	Elaborate form of Lucia; light [Latin]
Lucky	From a nickname for lucky person.
Lucy	English form of Lucia; light [Latin]
Luella	Variant of Louella; Lou + -ella
Lula	Diminutive of Louise; feminine form of Louis; famous in battle [Old German]
Lulu	Diminutive of names beginning with Lu-/Lou. Or pearl [Arabic]
Luna	The moon [Latin]
Luvinia	Variant of Lavinia; unknown meaning [Etruscan]
Lux	Light [Latin]

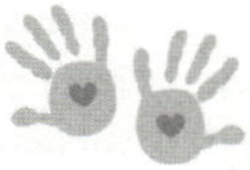

Lyda Variant of Lydia; woman from Lydia, Asia Minor [Greek]
Lydia Woman from Lydia, Asia Minor [Greek]
Lyla Variant of Layla; night [Arabic]
Lyn Variant of Lynn; from the lake [Welsh]. Or diminutive of Linda
Lynda Variant of Linda; beautiful [Spanish/Portuguese]; tender, soft [Old German]
Lyndsay Variant of Lindsay; from the surname; from Lindsay, Lincolnshire
Lyndsey Variant of Lindsay; from the surname; from Lindsay, Lincolnshire
Lynette Image/idol [Welsh]. Or diminutive of Lynn; of the lake [Welsh]
Lynn From the lake [Welsh]. Or diminutive of Linda
Lynne Variant of Lynn; from the lake [Welsh]. Or diminutive of Linda
Lynnette Variant of Lynette; Image/idol [Welsh]. Or diminutive of Lynn; of the lake [Welsh]
Lynsay Variant of Lindsay; from the surname; from Lindsay, Lincolnshire
Lynsey Variant of Lindsay; from the surname; from Lindsay, Lincolnshire
Lyric Lyric, song-like [Greek]
Lyssa Diminutive of Alyssa, a variant of Alicia; noble one [Greek]

M

Mabel Variant of Amabel; lovable one [Latin]
Mabella Elaborate form of Mabel; lovable one [Latin]
Mabelle Variant of Mabel; lovable one [Latin]. Also my beautiful one [French]
Mable Variant of Mabel; lovable one [Latin]
Macey Variant of Macy; from the surname; from Massy in France
Maci Variant of Macy; from the surname; from Massy in France
Macie Variant of Macy; from the surname; from Massy in France
Mackenzie From the surname; son of the handsome one [Gaelic]
Macy From the surname; from Massy in France
Madalyn Variant of Madeline/Magdalen; from the village of Magdala on the Sea of Galilee
Maddie Diminutive of Madeline. Or of Madison; from the surname; son of Maud
Maddison Variant of Madison; from the surname; son of Maud
Maddy Diminutive of Madeline. Or of Madison; from the surname; son of Maud
Madeleine French form of Magdalen; from the village of Magdala on the Sea of Galilee
Madelina Variant of Madeline/Magdalen; from the village of Magdala on the Sea of Galilee
Madeline English form of Magdalen; from the village of Magdala on the Sea of Galilee
Madelyn Variant of Madeline/Magdalen; from the village of Magdala on the Sea of Galilee
Madge Diminutive of Margaret; pearl [Greek/Sanskrit]
Madilyn Variant of Madeline/Magdalen; from the village of Magdala on the Sea of Galilee
Madison From the surname; son of Maud
Madisyn Variant of Madison; from the surname; son of Maud

Madlyn Variant of Madeline/Magdalen; from the village of Magdala on the Sea of Galilee
Madonna My lady [Italian]; title given to the Virgin Mary.
Madyson Variant of Madison; from the surname; son of Maud
Mae Variant of May; from the month named after the Roman goddess Maia.
Maegan Variant of Megan; Welsh dimutive of Margaret; pearl [Greek/Sanskrit]
Magda Diminutive of Magdalen; woman from the village of Magdala on the Sea of Galilee
Magdalen Woman from the village of Magdala on the Sea of Galilee
Magdalena Variant of Magdalen; woman from the village of Magdala on the Sea of Galilee
Magdalene Variant of Magdalen; woman from the village of Magdala on the Sea of Galilee
Maggie Diminutive of Margaret; pearl [Greek/Sanskrit]
Magnolia From the name of the flower
Mahala Weak; sick [Hebrew]
Mahalia Varaint of Mahala; weak; sick [Hebrew]
Maire Irish form of Mary; sea of sorrow; bitter; wished-for child [Greek]
Mairead Scots form of Margaret; pearl [Greek/Sanskrit]
Mairin Irish diminutive of Mary; sea of sorrow; bitter; wished-for child [Greek]
Maisie Scottish diminutive of Mairead/Margaret; pearl [Greek/Sanskrit]
Makayla Variant of Michaela; feminine form of Michael; who is like God? [Hebrew]
Makenna From the surname McKenna; born of fire [Gaelic]
Makenzie Variant of Mackenzie; from the surname; son of the handsome one [Gaelic]
Malandra Elaborate form of Andra/Andrea, feminine forms of Andrew; strong, manly [Greek]
Maleah Calm [Hawaian]. Or Hawaian form of Maria; sea of sorrow; wished-for child [Greek]
Malinda Variant of Melinda; Melanie/Melissa + -inda
Mallory From the surname; unfortunate [Norman French]
Malvina Smooth brow [Gaelic]
Mamie Diminutive of Margaret; pearl. Or of Mary; sea of sorrow; wished-for child [Greek]
Mandi Diminutive of Amanda; worthy of love [Latin]
Mandy Diminutive of Amanda; worthy of love [Latin]
Maralyn Variant of Marilyn; Mary + -lyn; sea of sorrow; bitter; wished-for child [Greek]
Marci Diminutive of Marcia; of the Roman god Mars
Marcia Feminine form of Marcius/Marcus; of the Roman god Mars
Marcie Diminutive of Marcia; of the Roman god Mars
Marcy Diminutive of Marcia; of the Roman god Mars
Margaret Pearl [Greek/Sanskrit]
Margaretha Dutch & German form of Margaret; pearl [Greek/Sanskrit]
Margaretta Latin form of Margaret; pearl [Greek/Sanskrit]
Margarita Greek form of Margaret; pearl [Greek/Sanskrit
Marge Diminutive of Margaret/Margerie; pearl [Greek/Sanskrit]
Margery Form of Margaret; pearl [Greek/Sanskrit]
Margie Diminutive of Margaret/Margerie; pearl [Greek/Sanskrit]
Margo Variant of Margot; French diminutive of Margaret; pearl [Greek/Sanskrit]
Margot French diminutive of Margaret; pearl [Greek/Sanskrit]
Marguerita Variant of Marguerite; pearl [Greek/Sanskrit]
Marguerite French form of Margaret; pearl [Greek/Sanskrit]

Maria Sea of sorrow; bitter; wished-for child [Greek]
Mariabella Maria + Bella
Mariah Variant of Maria; sea of sorrow; bitter; wished-for child [Greek]
Marian Variant of Marion, diminutive of Marie/Maria; sea of sorrow;wished-for child [Greek]
Marianna Maria + Anna
Marianne Diminutive of Marie/Maria; sea of sorrow; wished-for child [Greek]. Or Marie + Anne
Marie Variant of Maria; sea of sorrow; bitter; wished-for child [Greek]
Mariel Diminutive of Mary; sea of sorrow; bitter; wished-for child [Greek]
Marigold From the name of the flower; Mary + gold
Marilou Maria + Louise
Marilyn Mary + -lyn; sea of sorrow; bitter; wished-for child [Greek]
Marilynn Variant of Marilyn; Mary + -lyn; sea of sorrow; bitter; wished-for child [Greek]
Marina Of the sea [Latin]. Or feminine form of Marius; of the Roman god Mars
Marinda Diminutive of Mary; sea of sorrow [Greek]. Variant of Miranda; wonderful [Latin]
Marion French diminutive of Marie/Maria; sea of sorrow; bitter; wished-for child [Greek]
Maris Of the sea [Latin]
Marisa Maria + Luisa/Louise
Marissa Variant of Marisa; Maria + Luisa/Louise
Marje Diminutive of Marjorie; variant of Margaret/Margery; pearl [Greek/Sanskrit]
Marjorie Variant of Margaret/Margery; pearl [Greek/Sanskrit]
Marjory Variant of Margaret/Margery; pearl [Greek/Sanskrit]
Marla Diminutive of Marlene; Mary + Magdalen
Marlee Variant of Marley; from the surname; from a pleasant wood
Marleen Variant of Marlene; Mary + Magdalen
Marlena Variant of Marlene; Mary + Magdalen
Marlene Mary + Magdalen
Marley From the surname; from a pleasant wood
Marlin Variant of Marilyn; Mary + -lyn; sea of sorrow; bitter; wished-for child [Greek]
Marly Variant of Marley; from the surname; from a pleasant wood
Marlyn Variant of Marilyn; Mary + -lyn; sea of sorrow; bitter; wished-for child [Greek]
Marni Variant of Marnie; diminutive of Marina; of the sea [Latin]
Marnie Diminutive of Marina; of the sea [Latin]
Marsha Variant of Marcia; feminine form of Marcius/Marcus; of the Roman god Mars
Martha Lady; mistress [Aramaic]
Martie Diminutive of Martha or Martina
Martina Feminine form of Martin; of the Roman god Mars
Marva Feminine form of Marvin; famous friend; sea friend; from the sea fortress [Welsh]
Mary English form of Maria; sea of sorrow; bitter; wished-for child [Greek]
Maryann Mary + Ann
Maryanne Mary + Anne
Marybeth Mary + Beth
Marylou Mary + Lou/Louise
Marylu Variant of Marylou; Mary + Lou/Louise
Marylyn Variant of Marilyn; Mary + -lyn; sea of sorrow; bitter; wished-for child [Greek]

Mathilda	Variant of Matilda; strength in battle [Old German]
Matilda	Strength in battle [Old German]
Mattie	Diminutive of Matilda; strength in battle [Old German]
Matty	Diminutive of Matilda; strength in battle [Old German]
Maud	Form of Matilda; strength in battle [Old German]
Maude	Form of Matilda; strength in battle [Old German]
Maudie	Diminutive of Maud; form of Matilda; strength in battle [Old German]
Maura	Variant of Maire, Irish form of Mary; sea of sorrow; bitter; wished-for child [Greek]
Maureen	Irish diminutive of Mary; sea of sorrow; bitter; wished-for child [Greek]
Maurine	Diminutive of Mary; sea of sorrow; bitter; wished-for child [Greek]
Mavis	From an alternative name for the song thrush
Maxene	Variant of Maxine; feminine form of Max; greatest [Latin]
Maxime	French variant of Maxine; feminine form of Max; greatest [Latin]
Maxine	Feminine form of Max; greatest [Latin]
May	From the month named after the Roman goddess Maia. Diminutive of Mary, Mabel
Maya	Variant of Maia; from the Roman goddess. Or the Mayan people of America
Maybelle	Variant of Mabel; lovable one [Latin]
Maybelline	Diminutive of Mabel; lovable one [Latin]
Mayme	Diminutive of Margaret; pearl; sea of sorrow; bitter; wished-for child [Greek]
Mckayla	Variant of Michaela; feminine form of Michael; who is like God? [Hebrew]
Mckenna	From the surname; born of fire [Gaelic]
Mckenzie	Variant of Mackenzie; from the surname; son of the handsome one [Gaelic]
Meadow	Meadow
Meagan	Variant of Megan; Welsh dimutive of Margaret; pearl [Greek/Sanskrit]
Meaghan	Variant of Megan; Welsh dimutive of Margaret; pearl [Greek/Sanskrit]
Meg	Diminutive of Margaret; pearl [Greek/Sanskrit
Megan	Welsh dimutive of Margaret; pearl [Greek/Sanskrit]
Meghan	Variant of Megan; Welsh dimutive of Margaret; pearl [Greek/Sanskrit]
Mel	Diminutive of Melanie, Melissa etc.
Melanie	Dark; black [Latin]
Melantha	Mel + antha; dark flower
Melany	Variant of Melanie; dark; black [Latin]
Melba	From the Austrlain city, Melbourne
Melesina	Variant of Millicent; strong in labour [Old German]
Melina	Honey [Greek]. Or elaborate form of Mel- names
Melinda	Melanie/Melissa + -inda
Melisandre	French variant of Millicent; strong in labour [Old German]
Melissa	Bee [Greek]
Mellony	Variant of Melanie; dark; black [Latin]
Melody	Melody
Melva	Feminine form of Melvin/Melville; from a bad town [Norman French]
Memphis	Enduring and beautiful [Greek]
Mercia	Latin form of Mercy; from the virtue mercy
Mercy	From the virtue mercy

Meredith	Great lord; sea lord [Welsh]
Meriel	Variant of Muriel; bright sea [Gaelic]
Merilyn	Variant of Marilyn; Mary + -lyn; sea of sorrow; bitter; wished-for child [Greek]
Merla	Variant of Muriel; bright sea [Gaelic]
Merle	Variant of Muriel; bright sea [Gaelic]
Merletta	Diminutive of Merle/Muriel; bright sea [Gaelic]
Merlyn	Feminine form of Merlin; sea fortress [Gaelic]
Merrilyn	Variant of Marilyn; Mary + -lyn; sea of sorrow; bitter; wished-for child [Greek]
Merry	Merry; happy
Meryl	Variant of Muriel; bright sea [Gaelic]
Messiah	Deliverer; expected saviour [Aramaic]
Mia	Diminutive of Maria; sea of sorrow; bitter; wished-for child [Greek]. Or mine [Italian]
Mica	Diminutive of Michaela; feminine form of Michael; who is like God? [Hebrew]
Michaela	Feminine form of Michael; who is like God? [Hebrew]
Michele	Variant of Michelle; French feminine form of Michael; who is like God? [Hebrew]
Michelle	French feminine form of Michael; who is like God? [Hebrew]
Mickey	Diminutive of Michaela; feminine form of Michael; who is like God? [Hebrew]
Midge	Variant of Madge; diminutive of Margaret; pearl [Greek/Sanskrit]
Mikayla	Variant of Michaela; feminine form of Michael; who is like God? [Hebrew]
Mikhaila	Variant of Michaela; feminine form of Michael; who is like God? [Hebrew]
Mikki	Diminutive of Michaela; feminine form of Michael; who is like God? [Hebrew]
Mila	Gracious; dear [Slavic]
Mildred	Gentle strength [Old English]
Miley	Feminine diminutive of Miles; soldier [Latin].
Millicent	Strong in labour [Old German]
Millie	Diminutive of Midlred, Millicent etc.
Milly	Diminutive of Midlred, Millicent etc.
Mimi	Diminutive of Mary/Maria and other names beginning with M
Mina	Diminutive of Wilhelmina; feminine form of William; resolute protector [Old German]
Mindy	Diminutive of Melinda; Melanie/Melissa + -inda
Minerva	From the name of the Roman goddess; woman of intellect [Latin]
Minnie	Diminutive of Wilhelmina; feminine form of William; resolute protector [Old German]
Minta	Diminutive of Araminta; prayer and protection
Minty	Diminutive of Araminta; prayer and protection
Mirabelle	Wonderful; miraculous [Latin]
Miracle	Miracle, wonder
Miranda	Wonderful; admirable [Latin]
Mireille	Admire [French
Miriam	Sea of sorrow; bitter; wished-for child [Hebrew]
Missie	Diminutive of Melissa; bee [Greek]
Missy	Diminutive of Melissa; bee [Greek]
Misti	Variant of Misty; misty
Misty	Misty
Mo	Diminutive of Maureen; Irish diminutive of Mary; sea of sorrow; wished-for child

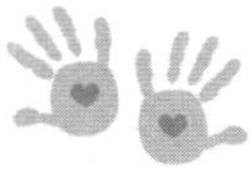

Modesty	From the virtue modesty
Moira	Variant of Maire, Irish form of Mary; sea of sorrow; bitter; wished-for child [Greek]
Mollie	Diminutive of Mary; sea of sorrow; bitter; wished-for child [Greek]
Molly	Diminutive of Mary; sea of sorrow; bitter; wished-for child [Greek]
Mona	My lady [Italian]. Or noble little one [Irish]
Monday	From the day of the week
Monica	Adviser [Latin]
Monique	French form of Monica; adviser [Latin]
Monna	Variant of Mona; my lady [Italian]. Or noble little one [Irish]
Montana	From the name of the US state; mountainous
Mora	Irish form of Mary; sea of sorrow; wished-for child [Greek]. Also great [Gaelic]
Morag	Little great one [Gaelic]. Or variant of Mary; sea of sorrow, wished for child [Greek]
Moreen	Diminutive of Mora. Or variant of Maureen; sea of sorrow, wished-for child [Greek]
Morgan	Sea defender [Welsh]
Morgana	Feminine form of Morgan; sea defender [Welsh]
Moriah	Seen by God [Hebrew]
Muriel	Bright sea [Gaelic]
Murphy	From the Irish surname; sea warrior [Irish]
Mya	Diminutive of Maria; sea of sorrow. wished-for child [Greek]. Or mine [Italian]
Myra	From myrrh [Latin]. Or anagram of Mary; sea of sorrow; wished-for child [Greek]
Myranda	Variant of Miranda; wonderful; admirable [Latin]
Myrtie	Diminutive of Myrtle; from the name of the shrub
Myrtle	From the name of the shrub

N

Nabila	Honourable; noble [Arabic]
Nadia	Variant of Nadya; hope [Slavic]
Nadine	Elaborate form of Nadia/Nadya; hope [Slavic]
Nadya	Hope [Slavic
Nahla	Drink of water [Arabic]
Nan	Diminutive of Ann; grace; favour [Hebrew]. Or diminutive of Nancy; chaste [Greek]
Nanette	Diminutive of Ann; grace; favour [Hebrew]
Nannie	Diminutive of Ann; grace; favour [Hebrew]
Nanny	Diminutive of Ann; grace; favour [Hebrew]
Naomi	Pleasantness [Hebrew]
Narcissa	Daffodil [Greek]
Narelle	Lake; little river [Australian Aboriginal]
Narissa	Variant of Nerissa; from the sea [Greek]

Nat	Diminutive of Natalia, Natalie etc.; birth of the Lord; Christmas Day [Latin]
Natalee	Variant ofNatalia; birth of the Lord; Christmas Day [Latin]
Natalia	Birth of the Lord; Christmas Day [Latin]
Natalie	Variant ofNatalia; birth of the Lord; Christmas Day [Latin]
Natalya	Variant ofNatalia; birth of the Lord; Christmas Day [Latin]
Natasha	Russian diminutive of Natalia; birth of the Lord; Christmas Day [Latin]
Nelda	Elaborate form of Nell; diminutive of Eleanor, Helen etc.
Nell	Diminutive of Eleanor, Helen etc.
Nelle	Variant of Nell; diminutive of Eleanor, Helen etc.
Nellie	Diminutive of Nell, Eleanor, Helen etc.
Nelly	Diminutive of Nell, Eleanor, Helen etc.
Nena	Variant of Nina; diminutive of names ending in -nina. Or little girl [Spanish]
Nerissa	From the sea [Greek]
Ness	Diminutive of Vanessa; a type of butterfly
Nessa	Diminutive of Vanessa; a type of butterfly
Netta	Diminutive of names ending in -netta
Nettie	Diminutive of names ending in -nette
Neva	Diminutive of Geneva, form of Genevieve; kinswoman [Germanic/Celtic]
Nevada	From the name of the US state; snow-capped [Spanish]
Nevaeh	Heaven, spelled backwards
Neve	English variant of Niamh; bright [Irish]
Nia	Welsh variant of Niamh; bright [Irish]. Or diminutive of names ending in -nia
Niamh	Bright [Irish]
Nichelle	Variant of Michelle; French feminine form of Michael; who is like God? [Hebrew]
Nichola	Feminine form of Nicholas; victory of the people [Greek]
Nichole	Feminine form of Nicholas; victory of the people [Greek]
Nicky	Diminutive of Nicola; victory of the people [Greek]
Nico	Diminutive of Nicola; victory of the people [Greek]
Nicola	Feminine form of Nicholas; victory of the people [Greek]
Nicole	Feminine form of Nicholas; victory of the people [Greek]
Nigella	Feminine form of Nigel, Latin form of Neil; cloud; champion [Gaelic].
Nikki	Diminutive of Nicola; victory of the people [Greek]
Nikole	Variant of Nicole; feminine form of Nicholas; victory of the people [Greek]
Nina	Diminutive of names ending in -nina. Or little girl [Spanish]
Nisha	Night [Hindi]
Nita	Diminutive of Anita; favour, grace [Hebrew]. And of other names ending in -nita
Noelene	Feminine diminutive of Noel; Christmas
Nona	Ninth [Latin]; 9th child or child born on 9th of the month
Nonie	Diminutive of Ione; violet flower [Greek]. Or of Nora; diminutive of Eleanor or Honora
Nora	Diminutive of Eleanor; light; radiance [Arabic]. Or of Honora; the virtue of honour
Norah	Diminutive of Eleanor; light; radiance [Arabic]. Or of Honora; the virtue of honour
Noreen	Diminutive of Nora/Eleanor/Honora
Norene	Diminutive of Nora/Eleanor/Honora
Norma	The rule; pattern; precept [Latin]. Feminine of Norman; from the north [Old German]

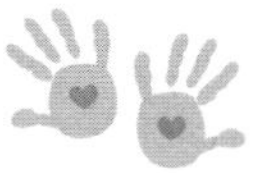

Normina Elaborate form of Norma; the rule; pattern; precept [Latin]. From the north
Nova New [Latin]
Nydia Nest [Latin]
Nyree English form of Ngaire; flaxen; blonde; pale [Maori]

O

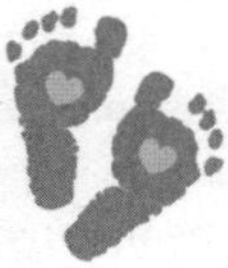

Ocean Ocean, sea
Oceana Ocean, sea
Octavia Eighth; 8th child, or one born on 8th of the month
Odelia Variant of Odilia; wealth; fortune [Old German]
Odilia Wealth; fortune [Old German]
Odell From the surname; from the woad hill
Odetta Variant of Odette; diminutive of Oda/Odila; wealth; fortune [Old German]
Odette Diminutive of Oda/Odila; wealth; fortune [Old German]
Olive Olive [Latin]. Or feminine form of Oliver; elf warrior [Old German]
Olivia Variant of Olive; olive. Or feminine form of Oliver; elf warrior [Old German]
Ollie Diminutive of Olive/Olivia; olive. Or feminine form of Oliver; elf warrior [Old German]
Olympia From Mount Olympus [Greek]
Olympie French variant of Olympia; from Mount Olympus [Greek]
Olyvia Variant of Olive; olive. Or feminine form of Oliver; elf warrior [Old German]
Oneida From the name of the Native American tribe; standing rock
Opal From the precious stone; jewel [Sanskrit]
Opaline Elaborate form of Opal; from the precious stone; jewel [Sanskrit]
Ophelia Help [Greek]
Ora To pray; one who prays [Latin]
Oralee Variant of Aurelie; golden [Latin]
Oralie Variant of Aurelie; golden [Latin]
Orinda Gold; golden one [Spanish]
Orpha Variant of Orpah; nape [Hebrew]
Ottilie Variant of Odilia; wealth; fortune [Old German]
Ottoline Diminutive of Ottilie/Odila; wealth; fortune [Old German]
Ourania Heavenly; one of the 9 muses, goddess of astronomy/astrology [Greek]

P

Paget	From the surname; little page
Paige	From the surname; page; servant
Paisley	From the surname; from the Scottish town Paisley
Pam	Diminutive of Pamela; sweetness [Greek]
Pamela	Sweetness [Greek]
Pamelia	Elaborate form of Pamela; sweetness [Greek]
Pamila	Variant of Pamela; sweetness [Greek]
Pansy	From the name of the flower
Parker	From the surname; park keeper
Parris	From the surname; from Paris, France
Pat	Diminutive of Patricia; noblewoman [Latin]
Patience	From the virtue patience [Latin]
Patrice	Variant of Patricia; noblewoman [Latin]
Patricia	Feminine form of Patrick; noblewoman [Latin]
Patsy	Diminutive of Patricia; noblewoman [Latin]
Patti	Diminutive of Patricia; noblewoman [Latin]. Or of Martha/Matty
Patty	Diminutive of Patricia; noblewoman [Latin]. Or of Martha/Matty
Paula	Feminine fom of Paul; humble one [Latin]
Pauleen	Variant of Pauline; humble one [Latin]
Paulene	Variant of Pauline; humble one [Latin]
Pauletta	Feminine diminutive of Paul; humble little one [Latin]
Paulina	Humble one [Latin]
Pauline	Humble one [Latin]
Payton	Variant of Peyton; from the English surname; from Paega's town [Old English]
Paz	Peace [Hebrew]
Pearl	Pearl
Pearlie	Diminutive of Pearl; pearl
Peg	Diminutive of Peggy/Margaret; pearl [Greek/Sanskrit]
Peggie	Diminutive of Margaret; pearl [Greek/Sanskrit]
Peggy	Diminutive of Meggy/Margaret; pearl [Greek/Sanskrit]
Pen	Diminutive of Penelope; duck; weaver [Greek]
Penelope	Duck; weaver [Greek]
Penny	Diminutive of Penelope; duck; weaver [Greek]
Peony	From the name of the flower
Persephone	Destroyer [Greek]
Peta	Feminine form of Peter; rock; stone [Greek]
Petra	Feminine form of Peter; rock; stone [Greek]. From the ancient city, Petra

Petrina	Feminine form of Peter; rock; stone [Greek]. From the ancient city, Petra
Petula	Meaning unknown; possibly pert or to attack
Petunia	From the name of the flower
Peyton	From the English surname; from Paega's town [Old English]
Phaedra	Bright [Greek]
Phebe	Variant of Phoebe; bright, pure one [Greek]
Phemie	Diminutive of Euphemia; speaks good omens [Greek]
Pheobe	Variant of Phoebe; bright, pure one [Greek]
Philadelphia	From the biblical city or the US city; brotherly love [Greek]
Philippa	Feminine form of Philip; friend of horses [Greek]
Phillis	Variant of Phyllis; foliage [Greek]
Philomena	Loved one [Greek]
Phoebe	Bright, pure one [Greek]
Phoenix	From the mythical bird reborn in fire [Greek]
Phyliss	Variant of Phyllis; foliage [Greek]
Phyllida	Of foliage [Greek]
Phyllis	Foliage [Greek]
Piety	From the virtie piety
Piper	One who plays the pipe or flute
Pippa	Diminutive of Philippa, feminine form of Philip; lover of horses [Greek]
Pleasance	Pleasant one [Old French]
Pollie	Variant of Mollie, diminutive of Mary; sea of sorrow; bitter; wished-for child [Greek]
Polly	Variant of Molly, diminutive of Mary; sea of sorrow; bitter; wished-for child [Greek]
Poppy	From the name of the flower
Porsche	From the name of the car company
Portia	From the Ancient Roman family name Porcius; pig/pork [Latin]
Posie	Diminutive of Josephine; he will add [Hebrew]. Or bunch of flowers [English]
Posy	Diminutive of Josephine; he will add [Hebrew]. Or bunch of flowers [English]
Praise	Praise
Precious	Precious; treasured
Presley	From the surname; from a priest clearing
Primrose	From the name of the flower
Primula	From the name of the flower family; the first [Latin]
Princess	Princess; ferminine of prince
Pris	Diminutive of Priscilla; of ancient family [Latin]
Priscilla	Of ancient family [Latin]
Prissy	Diminutive of Priscilla; of ancient family [Latin]
Pru	Diminutive of Prudence; prudence, caution, good judgement
Prudence	Prudence, caution, good judgement
Prue	Diminutive of Prudence; prudence, caution, good judgement
Prunella	From the name of the flower; plum [Latin]
Purdie	From the surname; by God [Norman French]

Q

Queen Woman; wife [Old English]
Queenie Diminutive of Queen; woman; wife [Old English]
Quinn From the Irish surname; descendant of the chief [Irish]

R

Rachael Variant of Rachel; ewe [Hebrew]
Racheal Variant of Rachel; ewe [Hebrew
Rachel Ewe [Hebrew]
Rachelle Variant of Rachel; ewe [Hebrew]
Rachyl Variant of Rachel; ewe [Hebrew]
Racquel Variant of Raquel; Spanish & Portuguese form of Rachel; ewe [Hebrew]
Rae Diminutive of Rachel; ewe [Hebrew]
Raelene Rae + -lene; diminutive of Rachel; ewe [Hebrew]
Raelyn Rae + -lyn; diminutive of Rachel; ewe [Hebrew]
Rain Rain
Rainbow Rainbow
Raine Queen; from la reine [French]. Or from Rain; rain
Ramona Feminine form of Ramon, Spanish form of Raymond; wise protector [Old German]
Rana Eye-catching one [Arabic]. King [Sanskrit]
Randi Diminutive of Miranda; wonderful; admirable [Latin]
Randy Diminutive of Miranda; wonderful; admirable [Latin]
Rania Diminutive of Ourania; heavenly [Greek]
Raquel Spanish & Portuguese form of Rachel; ewe [Hebrew]
Raven From the name of the bird
Ravenna Elaborate form of Raven. Or from the name of the Italian city
Raylene Ray + -lene; diminutive of Rachel; ewe [Hebrew]
Reagan From the Irish surname; impulsive [Irish]
Reanna Variant of Rhianna/Rhiannon; great queen [Welsh]
Reannon Variant of Rhiannon; great queen [Welsh]
Reba Diminutive of Rebecca; join [Hebrew]
Rebecca Join, tie [Hebrew]

Rebeccah Variant of Rebecca; join [Hebrew]

Rebekah Variant of Rebecca; join [Hebrew]

Reece Variant of Rhys; ardour; enthusiasm [Welsh]

Reene Variant of Renée; born again [Latin]. Or diminutive of names ending in -reen

Reenie Variant of Renée; born again [Latin]. Or diminutive of names ending in -reen

Reese Variant of Rhys; ardour; enthusiasm [Welsh]

Regan Little king [Gaelic]. Or variant of Reagan; impulsive

Regana Elaborate form of Regan; little king [Gaelic]. Or variant of Reagan; impulsive

Regena Variant of Regina; queen [Latin]

Regina Queen [Latin]

Reilly From a small stream; or courageous [Gaelic]; from a rye clearing [English]

Reinette Little queen [French]

Remington From the surname; from the settlement on the river bank [Old English]

Rena Latin form of Renée; born again [Latin].

Renée Born again; reborn [French/Latin]

Renee English form of Renée; born again [Latin].

Renie Variant of Renée; born again [Latin]

Renita Feminine form of Renatus; born again [Latin]

Retha Diminutive of Margaretha; pearl [Greek/Sanskrit]

Rhetta Feminine form of Rhett; from a Dutch surname; adviser

Rhianna Variant of Rhiannon; great queen [Welsh]

Rhiannon Great queen [Welsh]

Rhoda Rose [Greek]

Rhona Fair, blessed [Old English]; good spear [Welsh]; from the Hebridean island of Rona

Rhonda Good spear [Welsh]

Rhonwen Slender and fair [Welsh]

Rhys Ardour; enthusiasm [Welsh]

Rica Diminutive of Frederica and other names ending in -rica

Richardine Feminine form of Richard; brave power [Old German]

Richelle Feminine form of Richard; brave power [Old German]

Richmal Richard + Mary

Ricki Feminine diminutive of Richard

Rikki Feminine diminutive of Richard

Riley From a small stream; or courageous [Gaelic]; from a rye clearing [English]

Rilla Small brook; stream [Old German]

Rima White antelope [Arabic]

Rita Diminutive of Margherita; pearl [Greek/Sanskrit].

River River

Robbie Diminutive of Roberta; bright fame [old German]

Robena Diminutive of Roberta; bright fame [old German]

Roberta Feminine form of Robert; bright fame [Old German]

Robin Diminutive of Roberta; bright fame [old German]

Robina Diminutive of Roberta; bright fame [old German]

Robyn Diminutive of Roberta; bright fame [old German]

Robynne	Diminutive of Roberta; bright fame [old German]
Rochelle	From the name of the French city La Rochelle; little rock
Romaine	Roman woman [French]
Romayne	Variant of Romaine; Roman woman [French]
Romey	Diminutive of Rosemary; from the plant
Romy	Diminutive of Rosemary; from the plant
Rona	From the Scottish island Rona. Or fair, holy [Old English]. Or good spear [Welsh]
Ronda	Variant of Rhonda; good spear [Welsh]
Roni	Diminutive of Veronica; Latin variant of Berenice; bringing victory
Ronnette	Feminine form of Ronald; powerful counsellor [Old Norse]
Ronnie	Diminutive of Ronnette of Veronica
Ros	Diminutive of Rosalind, Rosamund and other names beginning with Ros-
Rosa	Latin form of Rose; from the name of the flower
Rosabel	Rosa + -bel; beautiful rose
Rosabella	Rosa + -bella; beautiful rose
Rosaleen	Variant of Rosaline/Rosalind; gentle horse [Old German]; beautiful rose [Latin]
Rosalie	Form of Rose; from the name of the flower
Rosalin	Variant of Rosalind; gentle horse [Old German]; beautiful rose [Latin]
Rosalind	Gentle horse [Old German]; beautiful rose [Latin]
Rosaline	Variant of Rosalind; gentle horse [Old German]; beautiful rose [Latin]
Rosalyn	Variant of Rosalind; gentle horse [Old German]; beautiful rose [Latin]
Rosalynne	Variant of Rosalind; gentle horse [Old German]; beautiful rose [Latin]
Rosamond	Variant of Rosamund; horse protector [Old German]; pure rose [Latin]
Rosamund	Horse protector [Old German]; pure rose [Latin]
Rosanna	Rose + Anna
Rosannah	Rose + Anna/Hannah
Rosanne	Rose + Anne
Rose	From the name of the flower
Roseann	Rose + Ann
Roseanne	Rose + Anne
Roselyn	Variant of Rosalyn/Rosalind; gentle horse [Old German]; beautiful rose [Latin]
Rosemarie	Variant of Rosemary; from the plant. Or Rose + Marie
Rosemary	From the plant. Or Rose + Mary
Rosie	Diminutive of Rose; from the flower
Roslyn	Variant of Rosalyn/Rosalind; gentle horse [Old German]; beautiful rose [Latin]
Rosy	Diminutive of Rose; from the flower
Rowan	From the name of the tree. Or from the surname; red-haired one [Gaelic]
Rowena	Unclear meaning; famous friend; slender; fair; good spear [Old German]
Rowina	Variant of Rowena; famous friend; slender; fair; good spear [Old German]
Roxana	Bright; dawn [Persian/Greek]
Roxane	Variant of Roxana; bright; dawn [Persian/Greek]
Roxanna	Variant of Roxana; bright; dawn [Persian/Greek]
Roxanne	Variant of Roxana; bright; dawn [Persian/Greek]
Roxie	Diminutive of Roxana; bright; dawn [Persian/Greek]

Roxy	Diminutive of Roxana; bright; dawn [Persian/Greek]
Roz	Diminutive of Rosalind, Rosamund and other names beginning with Ros-
Rozanne	Variant of Rosanne; Rose + Anne
Rubena	Behold a son [Hebrew]. Or like a ruby [Esperanto]
Rubina	Variant of Rubena; behold a son [Hebrew]. Or like a ruby [Esperanto]
Ruby	From the name of the precious stone; red
Rubey	Variant of Ruby; from the name of the precious stone; red
Ruth	Friend {Hebrew]
Ruthie	Diminutive of Ruth; friend [Hebrew]
Ryana	Feminine form of Ryan; from the surname; descendant of the little king
Ryann	Feminine form of Ryan; from the surname; descendant of the little king
Ryanne	Feminine form of Ryan; from the surname; descendant of the little king
Rylee	From a small stream; or courageous [Gaelic]; from a rye clearing [English]
Ryleigh	From a small stream; or courageous [Gaelic]; from a rye clearing [English]
Rylie	From a small stream; or courageous [Gaelic]; from a rye clearing [English]

S

Sable	Black [Slavic]
Sabra	Prickly pear [Hebrew]
Sabrina	From the Welsh name for the River Severn
Sabryna	Variant of Sabrina; from the Welsh name for the River Severn
Sadie	Diminutive of Sarah; lady; princess [Hebrew]
Saffron	From the name of the spice, or the colour [Arabic/Persian]
Sage	From the herb. Or wise person
Sal	Diminutive of Sally, a diminutive of Sarah; lady; princess [Hebrew]
Salena	Variant of Selina; heavenly [Latin]
Salina	Variant of Selina; heavenly [Latin]
Sallie	Diminutive of Sarah; lady; princess [Hebrew]
Sally	Diminutive of Sarah; lady; princess [Hebrew]
Salome	Peace [Hebrew]
Sam	Feminine form of Samuel; God has heard [Hebrew}] + -antha; flower [Greek]
Samantha	Feminine form of Samuel; God has heard [Hebrew}] + -antha; flower [Greek]
Samara	From the Biblical place name; watch mountain [Hebrew]
Sammi	Diminutive of Samantha; God has heard [Hebrew}] + -antha; flower [Greek]
Sammie	Diminutive of Samantha; God has heard [Hebrew}] + -antha; flower [Greek]
Sammy	Diminutive of Samantha; God has heard [Hebrew}] + -antha; flower [Greek]
Sandie	Diminutive of Sandra/Alexandra; the defender [Greek]
Sandra	Diminutive of Alexandra; the defender [Greek]

Sandy Diminutive of Sandra/Alexandra; the defender [Greek]
Santana Contraction of Santa Ana [Spanish]
Sapphire From the name of the blue gemstone
Sara Variant of Sarah; lady; princess [Hebrew]
Sarah Lady; princess [Hebrew]
Saranna Sarah + Anna
Sarina Diminutive of Sarah; lady; princess [Hebrew]. Or variant of Serena; tranquil [Latin]
Sasha Russian/Ukranian diminutive of Alexandra; defender [Greek]
Saskia Saxon; knife [Old German]
Savanna Variant of Savannah; grassy plain. Or from Savannah, Georgia, USA
Savannah Grassy plain. Or from Savannah, Georgia, USA
Scarlet From the colour. Or person who makes/sells scarlet clothes
Scarlett From the surname; person who makes/sells scarlet clothes
Seanna Feminine form of Sean, an Irish form of John; God is gracious [Hebrew]
Sebastiane Feminine form of Sebastian; from Sebaste, Asia Minor
Selby From the surname; from town of Selby; willow farm [Old Norse]
Selina Heavenly [Latin]
Selma Diminutive of Anselma; God's protection [Old German]
Senga Agnes spelled backwards; pure one [Greek]
September From the name of the month
Sequoia From the Californian trees [Cherokee]
Sera Variant of Sarah; lady; princess [Hebrew]. Or diminutive of Seraphina
Serafina Variant of Seraphina; fiery ones; Biblical order of angels [Hebrew]
Seraphina Fiery ones; Biblical order of angels [Hebrew]
Serena Serene; tranquil [Latin]
Serenity Tranquility [Latin]
Serina Variant of Serena; serene; tranquil [Latin]
Serrena Variant of Serena; serene; tranquil [Latin]
Shae Admirable; hawk-like [Gaelic]
Shaelyn Shae + -lyn; admirable; hawk-like [Gaelic]
Shana Variant of Shanna; from the Irish River Shannon
Shanelle Variant of Chanel; from the surname; pipe [French]; influenced by Coco Chanel
Shania Unknown meaning. Possibly on my way [Ojibwa]; or God is merciful [Hebrew]
Shanna From the Irish River Shannon
Shannah Variant of Shanna; from the Irish River Shannon
Shannen Variant of Shannon; from the name of the Irish river
Shannon From the name of the Irish river
Shantel Varient of Chantel/Chantal; stony; song [French]
Shari Diminutive of Sharon; Biblical place name; plain; from the shrub [Hebrew]
Sharise Variant of Charisse; from the French surname; grace; kindness [Greek]
Sharla Variant of Charla, a feminine form of Charles; warrior [Old German]
Sharleen Variant of Charlene; feminine diminutive of Charles; warrior [Old German]
Sharlene Variant of Charlene; feminine diminutive of Charles; warrior [Old German]
Sharmaine Variant of Charmaine; delight [Greek]

Sharon From the Biblical place name; plain; or from the shrub, rose of Sharon [Hebrew]
Sharona Form of Sharon; from the Biblical place name; plain; or from the shrub [Hebrew]
Sharron Variant of Sharon; from the Biblical place name; plain; or from the shrub [Hebrew]
Sharyl Variant of Cheryl; form of Cherie; darling [French]
Sharyn Variant of Sharon; from the Biblical place name; plain; or from the shrub [Hebrew]
Shauna Feminine form of Shaun/Sean/John; God is gracious [Hebrew]
Shavonne Anglicized form of Siobhan; a Gaelic form of Jane; God is gracious [Hebrew]
Shawna Feminine form of Shawn/Sean/John; God is gracious [Hebrew]
Shawnda Variant of Shonda; Shona + Rhonda
Shawnee Southern people [Algonquin]
Shaye Variant of Shae; admirable; hawk-like [Gaelic]
Shayla Variant of Sheila, a form of Cecilia; blind [Latin]
Sheba Oath [Hebrew].
Sheena Anglicized form of Sine, a Gaelic form of Jean; God is gracious [Hebrew]
Sheila Anglicized form of Sile, a Gealic form of Cecilia; blind [Latin]
Shelagh Variant of Sheila, a form of Cecilia; blind [Latin]
Shelby From the surname, a variant of Selby; from town of Selby; willow farm [Old Norse]
Shelia Variant of Sheila, a form of Cecilia; blind [Latin]
Shell Sea shell. Or diminutive of Michelle or Shelley
Shelley From the surname; from a clearing on a bank [Old English]
Shelly Variant of Shelley; from the surname; from a clearing on a bank [Old English]
Shena Variant of Sheena/Sine, a Gaelic form of Jean; God is gracious [Hebrew]
Sheree Variant of Sherry; descendant of the foal [Gaelic]. Influenced by Cherie [French]
Sherill Variant of Cheryl; form of Cherie; darling [French]
Sherilyn Variant of Cherilyn; Cheryl (darling) + -lyn
Sherisse Variant of Charisse; from the French surname; grace; kindness [Greek]
Sherri Variant of Sherry; descendant of the foal [Gaelic]. Influenced by Cherie [French]
Sherrie Variant of Sherry; descendant of the foal [Gaelic]. Influenced by Cherie; [French]
Sherry From the surname; descendant of the foal [Gaelic]. Influenced by Cherie;[French]
Sheryl Variant of Cheryl; form of Cherie; darling [French]
Shevaun Anglicized form of Siobhan; a Gaelic form of Jane; God is gracious [Hebrew]
Shevon Anglicized form of Siobhan; a Gaelic form of Jane; God is gracious [Hebrew]
Shirlee Variant of Shirley; from the surname; from a bright clearing [Old English]
Shirley From the surname; from a bright clearing [Old English]
Shona Scottish form of Joan; God is gracious [Hebrew]
Shonda Shona + Rhonda
Shyla Variant of Sheila, a form of Cecilia; blind [Latin]
Sibyl Prophetess [Greek]
Sibylla Latin form of Sibyl; prophetess [Greek]
Sidney From the surname; from a wide island [Old English]

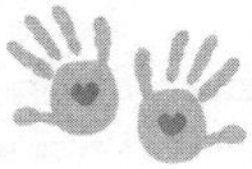

Sidra Of the stars; like a star [Urdu]
Siena Variant of Sienna; from the orange-red colour; from the Italian city
Sienna From the orange-red colour; from the Italian city
Sierra Mountain range [Spanish]

Silver	Silver; from the precious metal or colour
Silvia	Wood; forest [Latin]
Simone	French feminine form of Simon; he has heard [Hebrew]
Simonette	Diminutive of Simone; French feminine form of Simon; he has heard [Hebrew]
Sindy	Variant of Cindy, diminutive of Cynthia; woman of Kynthos [Greek]
Sinead	Irish form of Janet; God is gracious [Hebrew]
Sissie	Variant of Sissy; diminutive of Cecilia, Frances or Priscilla. Or of sister
Sissy	Diminutive of Cecilia, Frances or Priscilla. Or of sister
Sky	Sky
Skye	Variant of Sky. Or from the Isle of Skye, Scotland
Skylar	Variant of Skyler; scholar; from a Dutch surname
Skyler	Scholar; from a Dutch surname
Sloan	Variant of Sloane; from an Irish surname meaning little raider; warrior
Sloane	From an Irish surname meaning little raider; warrior
Snow	Snow
Soleil	Sun; sunny [French]
Sommer	Variant of Summer; summer
Sondra	Variant of Sandra; diminutive of Alexandra; defender [Greek]
Sonia	Variant of Sonya, Russian diminutive of Sophia; wisdom [Greek]
Sophia	Woman of wisdom [Greek]
Sophie	French form of Sophia; woman of wisdom [Greek]
Sophy	Variant of Sophy; or diminutive of Sophia; woman of wisdom [Greek]
Sorrel	From the name of the plant
Sparrow	From the name of the bird
Spirit	Spirit; breath
Spring	From the name of the season
Stacee	Variant of Stacy; diminutive of Anastasia. Or from the surname; fruitful [Greek]
Stacey	Variant of Stacy; diminutive of Anastasia. Or from the surname; fruitful [Greek]
Staci	Variant of Stacy; diminutive of Anastasia. Or from the surname; fruitful [Greek]
Stacia	Diminutive of Anastasia or Eustacia
Stacie	Variant of Stacy; diminutive of Anastasia. Or from the surname; fruitful [Greek]
Stacy	Diminutive of Anastasia. Or from the surname; fruitful [Greek]
Star	Star
Starla	Elaborate form of Star; star
Starr	Variant of Star; star
Stefani	Variant of Stephanie, feminine form of Stephen; crown, honour, reward [Greek]
Stella	Star [Latin]
Steph	Diminutive of Stepahnie; crown, honour, reward [Greek]
Stephani	Variant of Stephanie, feminine form of Stephen; crown, honour, reward [Greek]
Stephania	Feminine form of Stephen; crown, honour, reward [Greek]
Stephanie	Feminine form of Stephen; crown, honour, reward [Greek]
Stephany	Feminine form of Stephen; crown, honour, reward [Greek]
Stevie	Diminutive of Stephanie; crown, honour, reward [Greek]
Storm	Storm; tempest

Sue	Diminutive of Susan, Susanna etc; lily; rose [Hebrew]
Suellen	Susan + Ellen
Sukie	Diminutive of Susan, Susanna etc; lily; rose [Hebrew]
Summer	From the name of the season
Sunday	From the day of the week
Sunny	Sunny; cheerful; happy
Sunshine	Sunshine
Susan	Lily; rose [Hebrew]
Susana	Lily; rose [Hebrew]
Susanne	Variant of Susan/ Susana; lily; rose [Hebrew]
Susie	Diminutive of Susan, Susanna etc; lily; rose [Hebrew]
Suzan	Variant of Susan; lily; rose [Hebrew]
Suzanna	Variant of Susana; lily; rose [Hebrew]
Suzanne	Variant of Susan/ Susana; lily; rose [Hebrew]
Suzie	Diminutive of Susan, Susanna etc; lily; rose [Hebrew]
Sybella	Variant of Sibylla, Latin form of Sibyl; prophetess [Greek]
Sybil	Variant of Sibyl; prophetess [Greek]
Sydney	Variant of Sidney; from the English surname; from a wide island [Old English]
Sydnie	Variant of Sidney; from the English surname; from a wide island [Old English]
Sylvia	Variant of Silvia; wood; forest [Latin]
Sylvie	French variant of Silvia/Sylvia; wood; forest [Latin]
Symphony	Symphony

T

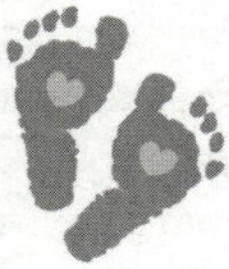

Tabatha	Variant of Tabitha; gazelle [Aramaic]
Tabby	Diminutive of Tabitha; gazelle [Aramaic]
Tabitha	Gazelle; gazelle-like [Aramaic]
Tahlia	Variant of Talia; from the name of the Australian town; near water [Aboriginal]
Taja	To name [Arabic]
Talia	From the name of the South Australian town; near water [Australian Aboriginal]
Tallulah	Leaping waters [Choctaw]. From the name of waterfalls in Georgia, USA
Tamar	Palm tree [Hebrew]
Tamara	Variant of Tamar; palm tree [Hebrew]
Tameka	Variant of Tamika; many beautiful children [Japanese]
Tamela	Tamara + Pamela
Tamika	Variant of Tamika; many beautiful children [Japanese]
Tammara	Variant of Tamar/Tamara; palm tree [Hebrew]
Tammi	Diminutive of Tamar/Tamara, Tamsin, Thomasina etc.

Tammie	Diminutive of Tamar/Tamara, Tamsin, Thomasina etc.
Tammy	Diminutive of Tamar/Tamara, Tamsin, Thomasina etc.
Tamra	Variant of Tamar/Tamara; palm tree [Hebrew]
Tamsen	Variant of Tamsin; diminutive of Thomasina, feminine form of Thomas; twin
Tamsin	Diminutive of Thomasina, feminine form of Thomas; twin [Aramaic]
Tamsyn	Variant of Tamsin; diminutive of Thomasina, feminine form of Thomas; twin
Tamzen	Variant of Tamsin; diminutive of Thomasina, feminine form of Thomas; twin
Tania	Variant of Tanya, Russian diminutive of Tatiana; from Roman family name
Tansy	From the name of the flower
Tanya	Russian diminutive of Tatiana; from Roman family name, Tatius; unknown meaning
Tanzi	Variant of Tansy; from the name of the flower
Tara	Anglicized form of Teamhair, the sacred hill of Irish high kings [Irish]
Tarah	Variant of Tara; the sacred hill of Irish high kings [Irish
Tarina	Elaborate form of Tara; the sacred hill of Irish high kings [Irish
Taryn	Feminine form of Tyrone; from the name of the Northern Irish county
Tasha	Diminutive of Natasha or Natalia; birth of the Lord; Christmas Day [Latin]
Tatiana	From Roman family name, Tatius; unknown meaning
Tatum	From the surname meaning Tata's home [Old English]
Tatyanna	Variant of Tatiana; from Roman family name, Tatius; unknown meaning
Tawnee	Variant of Tawny; from the light brown colour [French]
Tawnie	Variant of Tawny; from the light brown colour [French]
Tawny	From the light brown colour [French]
Tayla	Feminine form of Taylor; from the surname; tailor [Latin]
Tayler	Variant of Taylor; from the surname; tailor [Latin]
Taylor	From the surname; tailor [Latin]
Teaga	From an Irish surname; poet [Irish]
Teal	From the blue-green colour
Teale	Variant of Teal; from the blue-green colour
Temperance	Temperance, moderation
Tempest	Tempest; storm
Tera	Variant of Tara; the sacred hill of Irish high kings [Irish
Teresa	Variant of Theresa; summer; harvest [Greek]. Or from the Greek island Therasia
Teri	Feminine form of Terry; ruler of the people [Old German]. Diminutive of Theresa
Terra	Variant of Tara; the sacred hill of Irish high kings [Irish
Terri	Feminine form of Terry; ruler of the people [Old German]. Diminutive of Theresa
Terrie	Feminine form of Terry; ruler of the people [Old German]. Diminutive of Theresa
Terry	Ruler of the people [Old German]. Diminutive of Theresa; summer [Greek]
Tess	Diminutive of Theresa; summer; harvest [Greek]. Or from the Greek island Therasia
Tessa	Diminutive of Theresa; summer; harvest [Greek]. Or from the Greek island Therasia
Tessie	Diminutive of Theresa; summer; harvest [Greek]. Or from the Greek island Therasia
Thea	Diminutive of Dorothea or Theodora; gift of God [Greek]
Thelma	Invention of 19th century writer Marie Corelli; meaning unknown
Theodora	Feminine form of Theodore; gift of God [Greek]
Theresa	Summer; harvest [Greek]. Or from the Greek island Therasia

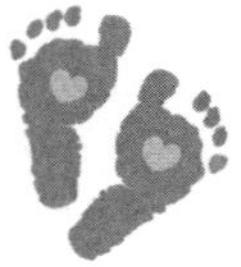

Therese Variant of Theresa; summer; harvest [Greek]. Or from the Greek island Therasia
Thomasina Feminine form of Thomas; twin [Aramaic]
Tia Diminutive of names ending in -tia
Tiana Diminutive of Christiana or Tatiana
Tianna Variant of Tiana; diminutive of Christiana or Tatiana
Tiara Tiara
Tibby Diminutive of Tabitha; gazelle [Aramaic]
Tierney Lord [Irish]
Tiffani Variant of Tiffany, a form of Theophania; manifestation of God [Greek]
Tiffany Form of Theophania; manifestation of God [Greek]
Tiffiny Variant of Tiffany, a form of Theophania; manifestation of God [Greek]
Tilda Diminutive of Matilda; strength in battle [Old German]
Tillie Diminutive of Matilda; strength in battle [Old German]
Tilly Diminutive of Matilda; strength in battle [Old German]
Tina Diminutive of names ending in -tina, e.g. Christina, Martina
Tisha Diminutive of Letitia or Latisha; happiness [Latin]
Toby A feminine form of Tobias; God is Good [Hebrew]
Tommie Diminutive of Thomasina, feminine form of Thomas; twin [Aramaic]
Toni Diminutive of Antonia; beautiful; priceless [Latin]
Tonia Diminutive of Antonia; beautiful; priceless [Latin]
Tonya Diminutive of Antonia; beautiful; priceless [Latin]
Topaz From the precious stone
Tori Diminutive of Victoria; victory {Latin]
Toria Diminutive of Victoria; victory {Latin]
Tory Diminutive of Victoria; victory {Latin]
Tottie Diminutive of Charlotte; warrior [Old German]
Totty Diminutive of Charlotte; warrior [Old German]
Tracee Variant of Tracy; from the surname; from a Norman place name [Norman French]
Tracey Variant of Tracy; from the surname; from a Norman place name [Norman French]
Traci Variant of Tracy; from the surname; from a Norman place name [Norman French]
Tracie Variant of Tracy; from the surname; from a Norman place name [Norman French]
Tracy From a Norman place name; domain of Thracius [Norman French]
Treasure Treasure; precious; valuable
Tresha Diminutive of Patricia; feminine form of Patrick; noblewoman [Latin]
Tricia Diminutive of Patricia; feminine form of Patrick; noblewoman [Latin]
Trina Diminutive of Katrina; Variant of Catriona, Gaelic form of Katherine; pure [Greek]
Trinity Trinity; three; Father, Son & Holy Ghost
Trish Diminutive of Patricia; feminine form of Patrick; noblewoman [Latin]
Trisha Diminutive of Patricia; feminine form of Patrick; noblewoman [Latin]
Trista Feminine form of Tristan, a French form of Drustan; tumultuous [Pictish]
Tristen Feminine form of Tristan, a French form of Drustan; tumultuous [Pictish]
Tristin Feminine form of Tristan, a French form of Drustan; tumultuous [Pictish]
Trix Diminutive of Beatrix; traveller [Latin]
Trixie Diminutive of Beatrix; traveller [Latin]

Trudi	Diminutive of Gertrude; strong spear [Old German]
Trudie	Diminutive of Gertrude; strong spear [Old German]
Trudy	Diminutive of Gertrude; strong spear [Old German]
Tulip	From the name of the flower
Twila	From twilight. Or star [French]
Twyla	Variant of Twila; From twilight. Or star [French]

U

Ula	Diminutive of Ursula; little bear [Latin]
Ulla	Diminutive of Ursula; little bear [Latin]
Ulyssa	Feminine variant of Ulysses; to hate [Greek]
Unice	Variant of Eunice; good victory [Greek]
Unique	Unique; one of a kind
Unity	Unity
Ursela	Variant of Ursula; little bear [Latin]
Ursula	Little bear [Latin]

V

Val	Diminutive of Valerie or Valentine
Valarie	Variant of Valerie; strong [Latin]
Valary	Variant of Valerie; strong [Latin]
Vale	wide river valley [Old English]
Valerie	From Roman family name Valerius; strong [Latin]
Valorie	Variant of Valerie; strong [Latin]
Vanessa	Type of butterfly
Velda	Powerful woman; ruler [Old German]
Velma	Variant of Wilma, a diminutive of Wilhelmina; resolute protector [Old German]
Velvet	Velvet
Venetia	Latin form of Gwyneth; fair; blessed [Welsh]. Or from the Italian city Venice
Vera	Faith [Russian]; truth [Latin]
Verena	Integrity; truth [Latin]
Verity	Verity, truth [Latin]

Verna Spring; green [Latin]. Or feminine form of Vernon; from the place of alder trees
Veronica Variant of Berenice; bringing victor.; influenced by vera icon. True image [Latin]
Veronique French form of Veronica; variant of Berenice; bringing victory. True image [Latin]
Veva Diminutive of Genevieve; kinswoman [Old German/Celtic]
Vi Diminutive of Violet; from the name of the flower
Vianne Diminutive of Vivianne; alive [Latin]. Or Vi + Anne
Vic Diminutive of Victoria; victory [Latin]
Vicki Diminutive of Victoria; victory [Latin]
Vickie Diminutive of Victoria; victory [Latin]
Vicky Diminutive of Victoria; victory [Latin]
Victoria Feminine form of Victor; victory, victor [Latin]
Vienna From the name of the Austrian city
Vikki Diminutive of Victoria; victory [Latin]
Viola The colour violet [Latin]
Violet From the name of the flower
Viona Variant of Fiona; fair [Gaelic]
Virgee Diminutive of Virginia; maid, virgin [Latin]
Virgie Diminutive of Virginia; maid, virgin [Latin]
Virginia Maid, virgin [Latin]
Virginie French form of Virginia; maid; virgin [Latin]
Vita Life [Latin]
Vivian Alive [Latin]
Viviana Latin form of Vivian; alive [Latin]
Vivianne Variant of Vivian; alive [Latin
Vivien Variant of Vivian; alive [Latin]
Vivienne French form of Vivian; alive [Latin]
Viviette Diminutive of Vivian; alive [Latin]
Vivyan Variant of Vivian; alive [Latin]
Vonda Variant of Wanda; woman of the Wend, a Slavic tribe

W

Wallis From the surname, a variant of Wallace; foreigner; Welsh [Norman French]
Wanda Woman of the Wend, a Slavic tribe
Wenda Variant of Wendy, a diminutive of Gwendolyn; fair, blessed [Welsh]
Wendolyn Variant of Gwendolyn; fair; blessed [Welsh]
Whitney From the surname; from the white island [Old English]
Wil Diminutive of Wilhelmina, feminine form of William; resolute protector [Old German]
Wilda Wild; untamed

Wilfreda Feminine form of Wilfred; desiring peace [Old English]
Wilhelmina Feminine form of William; resolute protector [Old German]
Willa Feminine form of William; resolute protector [Old German]
Willie Diminutive of Wilhelmina, feminine form of William; resolute protector [Old German]
Willow From the name of the tree
Willy Diminutive of Wilhelmina, feminine form of William; resolute protector [Old German]
Wilma Diminutive of Wilhelmina, feminine form of William; resolute protector [Old German]
Winifred Blessed peace [Welsh]
Winnie Diminutive of Winifred; blessed peace [Welsh]
Winnifred Variant of Winifred; blessed peace [Welsh]
Winona First-born daughter [Sioux]
Winter From the name of the season
Wisdom Wisdom
Wren From the name of the songbird
Wynona Variant of Winona; First-born daughter [Sioux]
Wynter Variant of Winter; from the name of the season

X

Xanthe Fair-haired one [Greek]
Xanthia Elaborate form of Xanthe; fair-haired one [Greek]
Xavia Feminine form of Xavier; the new house [Basque]
Xaviera Feminine form of Xavier; the new house [Basque]
Xenia Hospitable [Greek]

Y

Yara Small butterfly [Arabic]
Yasmin Variant of Jasmine; from the name of the plant [Persian]
Yasmine Variant of Jasmine; from the name of the plant [Persian]
Yazmin Variant of Jasmine; from the name of the plant [Persian]
Yolanda A form of Violet; from the name of the flower
Yolonda Variant of Yolanda; a form of Violet; from the name of the flower

Yvette French feminine form of Yves/Ivo; yew tree
Yvonne Feminine diminutive of Yves/Ivo; yew tree

Z

Zaina Variant of Zayna; beauty; grace [Arabic]
Zarah Blooming flower [Arabic]
Zandra Diminutive of Alexandra; the defender [Greek]
Zanna Diminutive of Susana; lily; rose [Hebrew]
Zara English form of Zaire/Zarah; blooming flower [Arabic]. Variant of Sarah
Zaria Variant of Zarah; blooming flower [Arabic]. OR from the Nigerian city Zaria
Zavanna Variant of Savannah; grassy plain. Or from Savannah, Georgia, USA
Zavia Variant of Xavia; feminine form of Xavier; the new house [Basque]
Zayna Beauty; grace [Arabic]
Zelda Diminutive of Griselda; grey battle [Old German]
Zelma Variant of Selma, diminutive of Anselma; God's protection [Old German]
Zena Variant of Xenia; hospitable [Greek]. Or diminutive of names ending with -sina.
Zenia Variant of Xenia; hospitable [Greek]. Or diminutive of names ending with -sinia.
Zenobia Force of Zeus [Greek]
Zinnia From the name of the flower
Zoe Life [Greek]
Zoë Variant of Zoe; life [Greek]
Zoey Variant of Zoe; life [Greek]
Zoie Variant of Zoe; life [Greek]
Zola Quiet; tranquil [Zulu]. Or earth [Latin]
Zowie Variant of Zoe; life [Greek]
Zulu From the southern African Zulu people

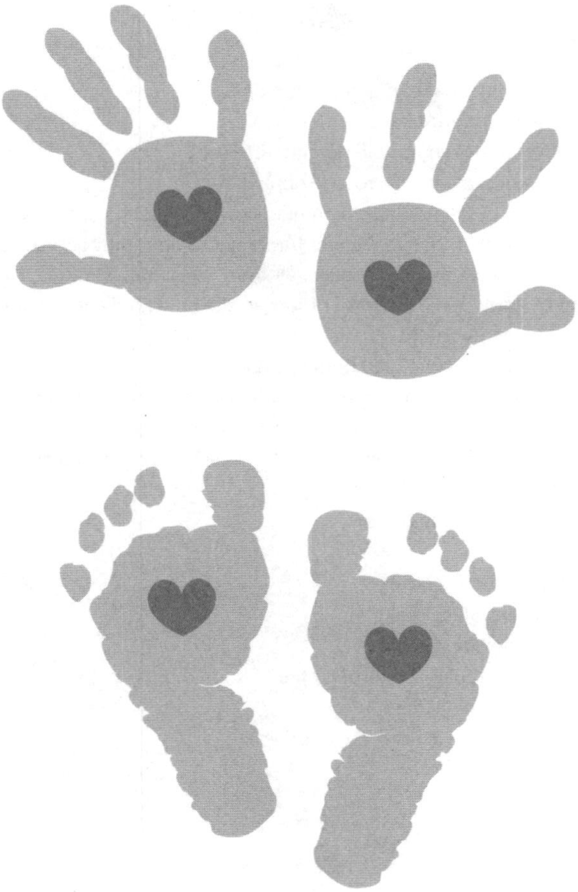

Boys

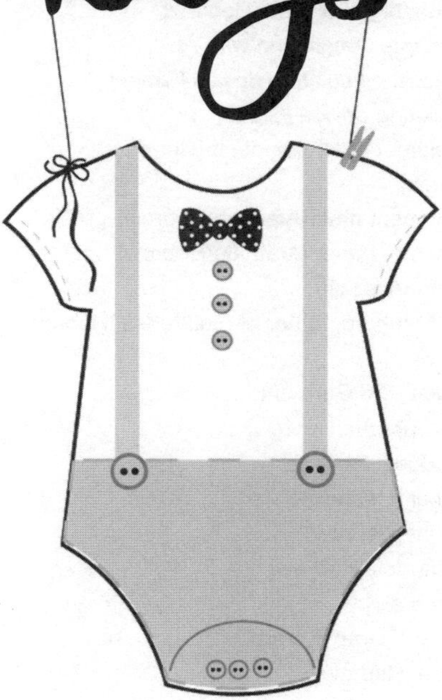

A

Aakil	Intelligent; smart [Hindi]
Aarav	Peaceful melody [Sanskrit]
Aaren	Variant of Aaron; high; exalted [Hebrew]
Aaron	High; exalted [Hebrew]
Aarron	Variant of Aaron; high; exalted [Hebrew]
Ab	Diminutive of names beginning with Ab-
Abacas	Variant of Abacus; calculating device [Greek]
Abacus	Abacus; calculating device [Greek]
Abalard	Variant of Abelard; noble; steadfast [German]
Aban	Little abbot [Irish]
Abbot	From the surname; father [Aramaic/Hebrew]
Abbott	From the surname; father [Aramaic/Hebrew]
Abdullah	Servant of Allah [Arabic]
Abe	Diminutive of Abraham; father of multitudes [Hebrew]
Abel	Breath [Hebrew]
Abelard	Noble; steadfast [Old German]
Abell	Variant of Abel; breath [Hebrew]
Abidan	My father is judge [Hebrew]
Abiel	God is my father [Hebrew]
Abner	My father is light [Hebrew]
Abraham	Father of multitudes [Hebrew]
Abram	High father [Hebrew]
Abraxas	Mythological god name [Persian]
Absalom	Father of peace [Hebrew]
Ace	From a nickname; highest rank; “top dog”
Acer	Botanical name for the maple tree [Latin]
Acker	From the surname; from the oak tree meadow [Old English]
Ad	Diminutive of names beginning with Ad-
Adair	From the surname derived from Edgar; wealthy spearsman [Old English]
Adam	Man [Hebrew]
Adamec	Czech variant of Adam; man [Hebrew]
Adams	From the surname; derived from Adam; man [Hebrew]
Addison	From the surname; son of Adam; man [Hebrew]
Aden	Variant of Aidan; little fire [Gaelic]
Adler	From the surname; eagle [German]

Adolph English form of Adolf, rare since WWII; noble wolf [Old German]
Adonis Lord [Greek]
Adrian English form of Hadrian; from Adria, Italy
Adriano Italian form of Adrian; from Adria
Adriel My help is God; flock of God [Hebrew]
Aed Variant of Aod; fire [Gaelic]
Aegidius Latin form of Giles; young goat [Greek/Latin]
Agassi From the surname [Armenian/Iranian]
Ahmed More commendable [Arabic]
Aidan Little fire [Gaelic]
Aiden Variant of Aidan; little fire [Gaelic]
Aidrian Variant of Adrian; English form of Hadrian; from Adria, Italy
Aimon Variant of Eamon, Irish form of Edmund; wealthy protector
Ainsley From the surname; from the woodland hermitage [Old English]
Aio Teacher; tutor [Italian]
Airlie From the Scottish surname
Aitken Scottish diminutive of Adam; man [Hebrew]
Akbar Praised [Arabic]
Al Diminutive of Alan, Albert and other names beginning with Al-
Alan Handsome; little rock [Breton]
Alaric All-powerful ruler; ruler of all [Old German]
Alasdair Scottish form of Alexander; the defender [Greek]
Alasdare Variant of Alasdair; Scottish form of Alexander; the defender [Greek]
Alastair Variant of Alasdair; Scottish form of Alexander; the defender [Greek]
Alban From Alba; white [Latin]
Albert Noble; bright [Old German]
Alberto Spanish & Portuguese form of Albert; noble; bright [Old German]
Albin Variant of Alban; from Alba; white [Latin]
Albus White [Latin]
Alcide French form of Heracles; glory of Hera [Greek]
Alcott From the surname; from the old cottage [Old English]
Alden From the surname; old friend [Old English]
Aldo Old and wise [Italian/Gereman
Aldous Old; wise [Old English]
Alec Diminutive of Alexander; the defender [Greek]
Alejandro Spanish form of Alexander; the defender [Greek]
Alessio Italian form of Alexis; the defender {Greek]
Alex Diminutive of Alexander; the defender [Greek]
Alexander The defender [Greek]
Alexis Helper; defender [Greek]
Alf Diminutive of Alfred; wise cousellor [Old English]
Alfie Diminutive of Alfred; elf counsel; wise couselor [Old English]
Alfonse French variant of Alfonso; noble; ready [Latin]
Alfonso Noble; ready [Latin]

Alfred	Elf cousel; wise cousellor [Old English]
Alfredo	Latin variant of Alfred; wise cousellor
Alfy	Diminutive of Alfred; wise cousellor [Old English]
Alger	From the surname; elf spear [Old English]
Algernon	From a norman nickname; has a moustache [Norman French]
Ali	Lofty; sublime [Arabic]. Or diminutive of names beginning with Al-
Alisdair	Variant of Alasdair; Scottish form of Alexander; the defender [Greek]
Alistair	Variant of Alasdair; Scottish form of Alexander; the defender [Greek]
Allan	Variant of Alan; handsome; little rock [Breton]
Allen	Variant of Alan; handsome; little rock [Breton]
Allyn	Variant of Alan; handsome; little rock [Breton]
Aloycius	A form of Louis; famous in battle [Old German]
Alpha	First letter of the Greek alphabet
Alphonso	Variant of Alfonso; noble and ready [Old German]
Alton	From the surname; from the town at the river source [Old English]
Alva	Variant of Alvah; His Highness [Hebrew]
Alvah	His Highness [Hebrew]
Alvaro	Cautious [German/Spanish]
Alvin	Elf friend; wise friend [Old English}
Amadeus	Lover of God [Latin]
Ambrose	Immortal [Greek]
Ambrosio	Latin variant of Ambrose; immortal [Greek]
Ambrosius	Variant form of Ambrose; immortal [Greek]
Amias	Loved [Latin]
Amir	Commander; prince [Arabic]. Tree-top [Hebrew]
Amit	Friend [Hebrew]; infinite [Sanskrit
Ammar	Devout; virtuous [Arabic]
Amory	Industrious [German]
Amos	Called [Hebrew]
Anatol	Variant of Anatole; from the east; rising sun [Greek]
Anatole	From the east; rising sun [Greek]
Anderson	From the surname; son of Andrew; strong; manly [Greek]
Andie	Diminutive of Andrew; strong; manly [Greek]
Andre	Variant of Andrew, from the French André; strong; manly [Greek]
André	French form of Andrew; strong, manly [Greek]
Andrei	Russian form of André/Andrew; strong; manly [Greek]
Andres	Spanish form of Andrew; strong; manly [Greek]
Andrew	Strong; manly [Greek]
Andy	Diminutive of Andrew; strong; manly [Greek]
Aneirin	Noble; golden [Welsh]
Aneurin	Variant of Aneirin; noble; golden [Welsh]
Angel	Angelic one; messenger [Greek]
Angus	One strength [Gaelic]
Ansel	Variant of Anselm; God's protection [Old German]

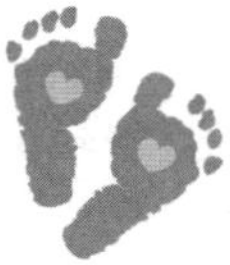

Anselm	God's protection [Old German]
Anson	From the surname; son of Agnes
Anthony	Meaning unknown; possibly priceless; handsome [Etruscan]
Antoine	French variant of Anthony; priceless; handsome [Etruscan]
Anton	Variant of Antony; meaning unknown; possibly priceless [Etruscan]
Antony	Older variant of Anthony; meaning unknown; possibly priceless [Etruscan]
Aod	Fire [Gaelic]
Archer	From the surname; archer; bowman
Archibald	Genuine; master; bold [Old German]
Archie	Diminutive of Archibald; genuine, master; bold [Old German]
Arden	From the surname; high [Celtic]
Ares	Ruin; bane [Greek]
Aric	Variant of Eric; always ruler [Old Norse]
Arian	Noble [Hindu/Sanskrit]. Masculine form of Ariana; most holy, immortal [Greek]
Ariel	Lion of God [Hebrew]
Arjun	Clear; bright; shining [Sanskrit/Hindu]
Arlen	From the surname; meaning unknown
Arlie	From the surname; eagle wood [Old English]
Arlo	Possibly from the Irish place name Aherlow; between two high lands [Irish]
Armand	Soldier [Old German]
Armani	Free man [Persian]
Arn	Diminutive of Arnold; eagle power [Old German]
Arnie	Diminutive of Arnold; eagle power [Old German]
Arnold	Eagle power [Old German]
Aron	Variant of Aaron; high; exalted [Hebrew]
Arron	Variant of Aaron; high; exalted [Hebrew]
Art	Diminutive of Arthur; bear; king [Celtic]. Or from Roman family name Artorius
Arthur	Bear; king [Celtic]. Or from Roman family name Artorius; unknown meaning
Arturo	Latin form of Arthur; bear; king [Celtic]. Or from Roman family name Artorius
Aryan	Noble [Hindu/Sanskrit]. Or masculine form of Ariana; most holy, immortal [Greek]
Asa	Healer [Hebrew]
Ash	From the name of the tree. Or diminutive of Ashley; ash meadow [Old English]
Asher	Happy; blessed [Hebrew]
Ashley	Ash meadow [Old English]
Ashton	From the surname; ash treee town [Old English]
Aston	From the surname; east town. Or noble stone [Old English]
Astor	Hawk [Occitan French]
Atticus	From Attica [Latin]
Atlas	From the god; not enduring [Greek]
Auberon	Variant of Aubrey; elf power; noble; bear like [Old German]
Aubrey	Elf power [Old German]
Audley	From the surname; Ealdgyd's clearing [Old English]
August	A form of Augustus; great [Latin]
Augustin	A form of Augustus; great [Latin]

Augustine Variant of Augustin/Augustus; great [Latin]
Augustus Great [Latin]
Austen Contraction of Augustine; great [Latin]
Austin Contraction of Augustine; great [Latin]
Austyn Contraction of Augustine; great [Latin]
Averill From the surname; boar battle [Old German]
Avery From the surname; powerful [Old German]
Avi My father [Hebrew]. Or diminutive of names beginning with Av-
Axel Father of peace [Old German]
Axl Variant of Axel; father of peace [Old German]
Axton Acca's stone or sword stone [Old English]
Ayaan Journey [Sanskrit]
Aydan Variant of Aidan; little fire [Gaelic]
Ayden Variant of Aidan; little fire [Gaelic]
Aylmer From the surname; variant of Elmer; noble; famous [Old English]
Azariah God has helped [Hebrew]

B

Bach From thesurname; one who lives near the brook [German]
Baden From the surname; son of Bade [German]
Baer Bear-like; bright [Old German]
Baez From the Spanish surname
Bahram Good-natured [Iranian]
Bailey From the surname; bailiff [Old English]
Bainbridge From the surname; near the bridge over the River Bain, Lincolnshire [Old English]
Baker From the surname; baker
Baku From the name of the city, capital of Azerbaijan
Baldassare Italian variant of Balthasar; God protects the king [Greek]
Baldric Brave ruler [Old German]
Baldwin Brave friend [Old German]
Balfour From the Scottish surname; village pasture [Gaelic]
Balin Mighty sword [Hindi]
Ballantine From the Scottish surname; place of worship [Gaelic]
Ballard From the surname; bald head [Old English]
Balliol From the Scottish surname; wall; fortification [Old French]
Balthasar God protects the king [Greek]
Barclay From a Scottish surname; birch wood [Old English]
Barnabas Son of the prophet; son of encouragement [Aramaic]

Barnaby	Variant of Barnabas; son od the prophet; son of encouragement [Aramaic]
Barney	Diminutive of Barnabas, Barnaby or Bernard
Baret	Variant of Barett; quarrelsome [Old English]; bear strength [Old German]
Barett	From the surname; quarrelsome [Old English]; bear strength [Old German]
Baron	Noble rank; or from the surname
Barrett	Variant of Barett; quarrelsome [Old English]; bear strength [Old German]
Barrie	Variant of Barry; head [Gaelic]
Barron	Variant of Baron; noble rank; or from the surname
Barry	Head [Gaelic]
Bart	Diminutive of Bartholomew; son of Talmai; furrowed [Hebrew]
Bartholomew	Son of Talmai; furrowed [Hebrew]
Basil	King [Greek]
Bastian	Diminutive of Sebastian; from Sebaste, Asia Minor [Latin]
Bastien	Diminutive of Sebastien; from Sebaste, Asia Minor [Latin]
Baxter	From the surname; baker [Old English]
Baylor	From the surname; one who delivers goods [Old English]
Baz	Diminutive of Barry; head [Gaelic]. Or of Basil; king [Greek]
Bazza	Diminutive of Barry; head [Gaelic]. Or of Basil; king [Greek]
Bear	Bear, the animal
Beal	Fair; handsome [Old French/English]
Beau	Beaitiful; handsome [French]
Beamont	From the surname; beautiful mountain [French]
Beauregard	From the surname; beautiful view [French]
Beckett	From the surname; from the stream/brook [Old English]
Beckham	From the surname; from the home by the stream [Old English]
Belisario	Swordsman [Greek]
Bellamy	From the surname; fine friend [Old French]
Ben	Son of the south; son of the right hand [Hebrew]. Blessed [Old English]
Benedict	Blessed [Old English]
Benj	Diminutive of Benjamin; son of the south; son of the right hand [Hebrew]
Benjamin	Son of the south; son of the right hand [Hebrew]
Benji	Diminutive of Benjamin; son of the south; son of the right hand [Hebrew]
Benjie	Diminutive of Benjamin; son of the south; son of the right hand [Hebrew]
Benjy	Diminutive of Benjamin; son of the south; son of the right hand [Hebrew]
Bennett	Variant of Benedict; blessed [Old English]
Bennie	Son of the south; son of the right hand. Or of Benedict, blessed [Old English}
Benny	Son of the south; son of the right hand Or of Benedict; blessed [Old English]
Benson	From the surname; son of Benedict; blessed [Old English]
Bentley	From the surname; from the bent grass woodland [Old English]
Benton	From the surname; from the bent grass enclosure [Old English]
Bernard	Brave; strong as a bear [Old German]
Bernardo	Latin form of Bernard; brave; strong as a bear [Old German]
Bernie	Diminutive of Bernard; brave; strong as a bear [Old German]
Berny	Diminutive of Bernard; brave; strong as a bear [Old German]

Berry	Variant of Barry; head [Gaelic]
Bert	Diminutive of Albert, Herbert and other names ending in -bert; bright [Old German]
Bertie	Diminutive of Albert, Herbert and other names ending in -bert; bright [Old German]
Bertram	Bright raven [Old German]
Bertrand	Bright shield [Old German]
Beverly	From the surname; from the city of Beverly; beaver stream [Old English]
Bevis	From the surname; from Beavais, France
Biff	From a nickname; to hit, punch
Bilal	Refreshing; wetting [Arabic]
Bill	Diminutive of William; resolute protector [Old German]
Billie	Diminutive of William; resolute protector [Old German]
Billy	Diminutive of William; resolute protector [Old German]
Binek	White [Czech]
Bing	From a nickname; from a hollow [Old English]. Or soldier [Chinese]
Bishop	From the surname; bishop; overseer [Greek]
Bjorn	Bear [Swedish]
Blaine	From a Scottish surname; yellow; yellow-haired [Gaelic]
Blair	From the Scottish surname; field; battlefield [Gaelic]
Blaise	Lisping one [Latin]
Blake	From the surname; black; or pale [Old English]
Blakeley	From the surname; from a dark wood; dark clearing [Old English]
Blaze	Variant of Blaise; lisping one [Latin]. Or blaze
Blythe	From the surname; cheerful [Old English]
Bo	From a Norse nickname; to live [Old Norse]
Boaz	Swiftness [Hebrew]
Bob	Diminutive of Robert; bright fame [Old German]
Bobbie	Diminutive of Robert; bright fame [Old German]
Bobby	Diminutive of Robert; bright fame [Old German]
Bodhi	Awakening; enlightenment [Sanskrit]
Bodie	Variant of Bodhi; awakening; enlightenment [Sanskrit]. Messenger [Old Norse]
Bogdan	God given [Slavic]
Bolivar	From the surname; from the mill at the river bank [Basque]
Bolton	From the surname; from the English town; from the enclosure/field [Old English]
Bond	From the surname; bondsman; peasant farmer [Old English]
Bono	From the Italian surname; good [Latin]
Booker	From the surname; maker of books
Boone	Blessing; or from the surname [English/French]
Boris	Short; wolf; snow leapard [Turkic]
Bowen	Son of Owen [Welsh]
Bowie	From the surname; from a nickname for fair-haired/yellow-haired person [Gaelic]
Boyce	From the surname; from the wood [French]
Boyd	From the Scottish surname; from the Isle of Bute
Brad	Diminutive of names beginning with Brad-
Braden	From the Irish surname; salmon [Irish]

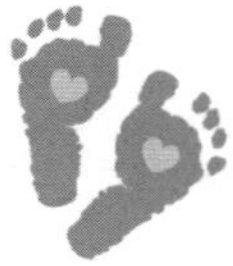

Bradford	From the surname; from Bradford; broad ford [Old English]
Bradley	From the surname; from a broad clearing [Old English]
Brady	From the Irish surname; broad chested [Gaelic]
Braeden	Variant of Braden; from the Irish surname; salmon [Irish]
Braiden	Variant of Braden; from the Irish surname; salmon [Irish]
Braidy	Variant of Brady; from the Irish surname; broad chested [Gaelic]
Braith	Freckled; speckled; black and white; red and white [Gaelic]
Bram	Diminutive of Abraham; father of multitudes [Hebrew]
Brand	Variant of Brant; surname; fire; sword [Old Norse]
Branden	Variant of Brandon; from the surname; from the broom-covered hill [Old English]
Brando	Italian variant of Brant/Brand; from the surname; fire; sword [Old Norse]
Brandon	From the surname; from the broom-covered hill [Old English]
Brandt	Variant of Brant; from the surname; fire; sword [Old Norse]
Brannon	From the Irish surname; raven
Branson	From the surname; son of the fire/sword [Old Norse]
Brant	From the surname; fire; sword [Old Norse]
Brantley	From the surname; fire; sword [Old Norse]
Brax	Variant of Brock; badger
Braxton	From the surname; from Bracca's town
Brayden	Variant of Braden; from the Irish surname; salmon [Irish]
Braylen	Brayden + Jaylen
Breck	Speckled [Gaelic]
Breckan	Elaborate form of Breck; speckled [Gaelic]
Breckin	Elaborate form of Breck; speckled [Gaelic]
Brendan	Prince [Welsh/Irish Gaelic]
Brenden	Variant of Brendan; prince [Welsh/Irish Gaelic]
Brendon	Variant of Brendan; prince [Welsh/Irish Gaelic]
Brennan	From the surname; raindrop; moisture
Brent	From the surname; hill [Celtic]
Brentley	Brent + ley
Brenton	From the surname; from Bryni's town; fire
Bret	Variant of Brett, from the surname; Breton; from Brittany
Brett	From the surname; Breton; from Brittany
Brian	High; noble [Gaelic]
Briar	Briar; thorny patch
Brice	Speckled one [Gaulish]
Bridger	From the surname; one who lives near a bridge
Briggs	From the surname; a variant of Bridges; one who lives near a bridge [Old English]
Brigham	From the surname; from the bridge village/settlement
Brighton	From the name of the English town; bright town
Brion	Variant of Brian; high; noble [Gaelic]
Briscoe	From the surname; birch wood [Old Norse]
Bristol	From the surname/place name; English city; site of the bridge
Britton	From the surname; Celtic inhabitant of Britain or Brittany.

Brixton	From the place name or surname
Brock	From the surname; badger [Old English]
Broderick	Brother [Old Norse]
Brodie	From the Scottish surname derived from the place name; ditch; mire [Gaelic]
Brody	From the Scottish surname derived from the place name; ditch; mire [Gaelic]
Brogan	From the Irish surname; small shoe [Irish]
Bronte	From the Irish surname; bestower [Gaelic]. Or thunder [Greek]
Brook	From the surname; one who lives near a brook
Brooklyn	From the area of New York City
Brooks	Variant of Brook; from the surname; one who lives near a brook
Bruce	From the Scottish surname; from Brix, France [Norman French]
Bruno	Brown; armour protection [Old German]
Bryan	Variant of Brian; high; noble [Gaelic]
Bryant	From the surname derived from Brian; high; noble [Gaelic]
Bryce	Variant of Brice; speckled one [Gaulish]
Brycen	Variant of Bryson; from the surname; son of Brice; son of the speckled one
Bryn	Hill, mound [Welsh]
Bryon	Variant of Brian; high; noble [Gaelic]
Bryson	From the surname; son of Brice; son of the speckled one
Bubba	From US southern nickname
Buck	From a nickname; male deer
Bud	Diminutive of Buddy; from a nickname; friend; brother
Buddy	From a nickname; friend; brother
Burke	From the surname; from the fortress/town [Old English]
Burleigh	From the surname; from the manor's meadow [Old English]
Burley	Variant of Burleigh; from the surname; from the manor's meadow [Old English]
Burt	Diminutive of Burton; fortified town [Old English]. Or of names ending in -bert
Burton	From a surname; fortified town [Old English]
Buster	From a nickname; one who breaks things
Byrne	From the Irish surname; descendant of Bran; raven [Irish]
Byron	From the surname; from the olace of the cowsheds [Old Englsih]
Bysshe	Variant of the surname Bush; one who lives near a bush

C

Cabe	Diminutive of names beginning with Cab-
Cabel	Variant of cable; rope
Cable	Cable; rope
Cabot	From the surname; to sail [French]

Cadan Vaiant of Caden; spirit of battle [Gaelic]. Or friend; companion [Arabic]
Caddock From Cadoc; eager for war [Welsh]
Cade From the surname derived from a nickname; round [Old English]
Cadell From the surname; battle [Welsh]
Caden From the Irish surname; spirit of battle [Gaelic]. Or friend; companion [Arabic]
Cadmus One who excells [Greek]
Cadogan Honour in battle [Welsh]
Cador Battle king [Cornish]
Caelan Slender [Gaelic]
Cagney From the Irish surname; tribute [Irish]
Cahir Variant of Cathair; man of battle [Irish]
Cai Variant of Caius, Cairo or Kai
Caiden Variant of Caden; spirit of Battle [Gaelic]. Or friend; companion [Arabic]
Cailean Variant of Calum; Scottish form of Columba; dove [Latin]. Or young dog [Gaelic]
Cain Acquired; possessed [Hebrew]
Caio Variant of Caius; rejoice [Latin]
Cairn Mound of stones [Gaelic]
Cairo From the Egyptian city; victorious [Arabic]
Caius Rejoice [Latin]
Cal Diminutive of names beginning with Cal-
Calbert Calf-herder [Old English]
Cale Diminutive of Caleb; dog; or whole heart [Hebrew]
Caleb Dog; or whole heart [Hebrew]
Caledon From Caledon; hard, rocky land [Irish]. Masculine variant of Caledonia [Latin]
Calum Scottish form of Columba; dove [Latin]
Callahan From the surname; bright headed [Irish]
Callan Variant of Caelan; slender [Gaelic]
Callum Variant of Calum; Scottish form of Columba; dove [Latin]
Calton From the surname; from the calf-farm [Latin]
Calvin From the French surname Chauvin; bald [Latin]
Cam Diminutive of Cameron; from the Scottish surname; crooked nose [Gaelic]
Camden From the place name/area of London; enclosed valley [Old English]
Cameron From the Scottish surname; crooked nose [Gaelic]
Camille Masculine form of Camilla; unblemished virgin; or religious attendant [Latin]
Camilo Masculine form of Camilla; unblemished virgin; or religious attendant [Latin]
Camron Variant of Cameron; from the Scottish surname; crooked nose [Gaelic]
Canaan From the Biblical place name
Canady Variant of Kennedy; from the Irish surname; armoured head [Gaelic]
Cannon Cannon; or from the surname Canon, a church official
Caradoc Beloved; amiable [Welsh]
Carew From the surname; from the hill fort [Welsh]
Carey From the Irish surname; black [Irish]
Carl German form of Charles; warrior [Old German]
Carleton Variant of Charlton; from a settlement/village of free men [Old English]

Carlisle	From the surname; from the English city of Carlisle; fortress of Lugus [Latin]
Carlitos	Spanish diminutive of Charles; warrior [Old German]
Carlos	Spanish form of Charles; warrior [Old German]
Carlton	Variant of Charlton; from a settlement/village of free men [Old English]
Carlyle	Variant of Carlisle; from the English city of Carlisle; fortress of Lugus [Latin]
Carmelo	Cultivated land [Spanish/Hebrew]
Carmichael	From the Scottish surname; Michael's fort [Celtic]
Carmine	From the name of the bright red colour
Carmino	Variant of Carmine; from the name of the bright red colour
Carnelian	From the name of the gemstone
Carran	From the Irish surname; little spear [Irish]
Carson	Descendant of the marsh [Old English]; from the fort [Welsh]; the rock [Gaelic]
Carter	From the surname; cart user/worker
Carver	From the surname; wood carver
Cary	Variant of Carey; from the Irish surname; black [Irish]
Case	Case. Or short form of Casey; from the surname; vigilant [Irish]
Casey	From the surname; vigilant [Irish]
Cash	From the surname; box-maker [French]
Casimir	Destroyer of fame/prestige/peace; proclaims peace [Slavic]
Cass	Diminutive of Cassidy and other names beginning with Cass-
Cassidy	From the Irish surname; curly-haired [Irish]
Cassius	From the Roman family name; vain; empty [Latin]
Castiel	My cover is God; shield of God [Hebrew]
Cathair	Man of battle [Irish]
Cato	All-knowing [Latin]
Catoe	Variant of Cato; all-knowing [Latin]
Cavan	From the name of the Irish county; hollow. Gentle, beautiful [Irish]
Cavanaugh	From the Irish surname; born handsome [Irish]
Cayden	Variant of Caden. Spirit of Battle [Gaelic]. Or friend; companion [Arabic]
Cael	Slender [Gaelic]
Calder	From the surname; rocky water [Old English]
Campbell	From the surname; crooked mouth [Gaelic]
Canyon	Canyon
Carsen	Variant of Carson; son of the marsh dweller [Old English]
Carson	From the surname; son of the marsh dweller [Old English]
Carver	From the surname; wood carver
Cason	Invented name to rhyme with Kason, Jason, Mason etc
Casper	Dutch form of Jasper; treasurer [Persian]
Caspian	From the name of the Caspian Sea
Ceasar	From the Roman family name; long-haired [Latin]
Cesar	Variant of Ceasar; from the Roman family name; long-haired [Latin]
Cecil	From a Roman family name; blind [Latin]
Cedar	From the name of the tree [Greek]
Cedric	Love [Celtic]

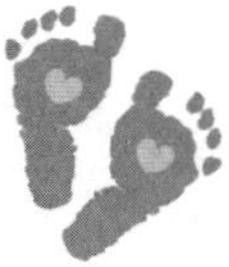

Celeste	Heavenly [Latin]
Chad	Battle [Welsh]
Chadwick	From the surname; settlement of Chad; battle [Welsh]
Chaim	Life [Hebrew]
Chance	Diminutive of the surname Chauncey; luck; fortune
Chandler	From the surname; candle seller [Old French]
Channing	From the surname; little wolf cub
Charles	Man; warrior [Old German]
Charlie	Diminutive of Charles; man; warrior [Old German]
Charley	Diminutive of Charles; man; warrior [Old German]
Charlton	From the surname; from a settlement/village of free men [Old English]
Chas	Diminutive of Charles; man; warrior [Old German]
Chace	Variant of Chase; from the surname; huntsman [Old English]
Chase	From the surname; huntsman [Old English]
Chauncey	From the Norman surname; luck; fortune; chance
Chaz	Diminutive of Charles; man; warrior [Old German]
Cherokee	People of a diferent speech [Creek/Native American]
Chesley	From the surname; from the meadow camp [Old English]
Chester	From the surname; from city of Chester; fortress [Latin]
Chet	Diminutive of Chester; from the surname; from city of Chester; fortress [Latin]
Chevy	Diminutive of Chevalier; knight; horseman [French]
Cheyenne	From the Native American people; red speakers [Dakota/Native American]
Chip	Diminutive of Charles; warrior [Old German]. Or Christopher; bearing Christ
Chosen	Chosen
Chris	Diminutive of Christian, Christopher etc.
Christian	Christian
Christmas	From the Christian festival
Christopher	Bearing Christ; carrying Christ [Greek]
Chuck	Diminutive of Charles; warrior [Old German]
Cian	Ancient [Gaelic]
Ciaran	Little dark one [Gaelic]
Cillian	Little church; little strife [Irish]
Ciprian	Variant of Cyprian; man of Cyprus
Ciro	Italian variant of Cyrus; far-sighted; young [Greek]
Clair	French form of Clarus; clear; famous [Latin]
Clancey	From the Irish surname; red warrior [Gaelic]
Clarence	Man from Clare, Suffolk, England
Clark	From the surname; cleric; scribe [Old English]
Claud	Variant of Claude; from the Roman famiy name; lame [Latin]
Claude	From the Roman family name; lame [Latin]
Clay	Man who works with clay. Diminutive of Clayton; from the clay settlement
Clayton	From the surname; from the place of good clay [Old English]
Clem	Diminutive of Clement; merciful [Latin]
Clement	Merciful [Latin]

Cletis	Variant of Cletus; diminutive of Analectus; invoked [Greek]
Cletus	Diminutive of Analectus; involed [Greek]
Cleve	Diminutive of Cleveland; from the surname; from hilly land [Old English]
Cleveland	From the surname; from hilly land [Old English]
Cliff	Diminutive of Clifford or Clifton
Clifford	From the surname; from the ford by the cliff [Old English]
Clifton	From the surname; settlement/town by the cliff [Old English]
Cint	Diminutive of Clinton; from settlement by the River Glyme [Old English]
Clinton	From the surname; from settlement by the River Glyme [Old English]
Clive	From the surname; one who lives near a cliff {Old English]
Clyde	From the name of the Scottish river;
Coby	Diminutive of Jacob; supplanter [Hebrew]
Codie	Variant of Cody; from the surname; helpful [Irish]
Cody	From the Irish surname; helpful [Irish]
Coen	Variant of Cohen, Jewish surname; priest [Hebrew]
Cohen	From the Jewish surname; priest [Hebrew]
Colbert	From the surname; bright helmet [Old German]
Colby	From the surname; dark town; coal town [Old Norse]
Cole	From the surname; charcoal; one who is dark-featured [Old English]
Coleman	From the surname; from a diminutive of Columba; dove [Latin]
Coleridge	From the surname; from the ridge where charcoal is burned [Old English
Colin	English form of Cailean/Calum, Scottish form of Columba; dove [Latin].
Collier	From the surname; coal miner
Collin	Variant of Colin; dove [Latin]. Diminutive of Nicholas; victory of the people [Greek]
Colt	From the surname; or colt; young male horse
Colten	Variant of Colton; from the surname; from Cola's town; from colt-breeding town
Colton	From the surname; from Cola's town; from colt-breeding town
Conall	Strong wolf [Gaelic]
Conn	Diminutive of name beginning with Con-
Connell	Variant of Conall; strong wolf;
Conner	Variant of Conor; dog-lover; wolf-lover [Gaelic]
Connor	Variant of Conor; dog-lover; wolf-lover [Gaelic]
Conor	Dog-lover; wolf-lover [Gaelic]
Conrad	Brave cousellor [Old German]
Constant	Constant; steadfast [Latin]
Constantine	Constant; steadfast [Latin]
Conway	From the surname; of the holy water [Welsh]
Cooper	From the surname; barrel maker [Old English]
Corbin	From the surname; raven; one with black hair [French]
Cordell	From the surname; maker/seller of cord [Old English]
Corey	From the surname; hollow-dweller; spear
Cormac	Son of the raven; wheel; charioteer [Irish]
Cornelius	From the Roman family name; of the horn [Latin]
Cornell	From the surname; derived from Cornelius; of the horn [Latin]

Cortney	Variant of Courtney; from the surname; short-nose [Norman French]
Corwin	From the surname; leather worker/seller [French/Spanish]
Cory	Variant of Corey; from the surname; hollow-dweller; spear
Cosmo	Variant of the Italian Cosimo; order; decency [Greek]
Coty	Variant of Cody; from the surname; helpful [Irish]
Courtney	From the surname; short-nose [Norman French]
Coy	From the surname; shy, coy [Old English]
Craig	From the Scottish surname; living near a hill/crag [Gaelic]
Crawford	From the surname; from the crow ford [Old English]
Cree	From the Native American tribe in Canada
Creed	Creed; belief system
Creighton	From the surname; from the border town [Gaelic]
Crew	Crew
Crispin	Curly-haired [Latin]
Cristiano	Christian [Italian & Portuguese]
Cristobal	Spanish form of Chritopher; bearing Christ; carrying Christ [Greek]
Crofton	From the surname; from a town with an eclosed field [Old English]
Cruz	Cross [Spanish]
Cullen	From Cologne, Germany; colony [Latin]. Or young dog; dove [Gaelic]
Curt	Variant of Kurt; diminutive of Conrad; brave counsellor Diminutive of Curtis
Cuthbert	Famous; bright [Old English]
Cy	Diminutive of Cyrus; far-sighted; young [Greek]. Or of Cyril; lord [Greek]
Cyan	From the name of the green-blue colour [Greek]
Cyprian	Man of Cyprus
Cyril	Lord [Greek]
Cyrus	Far-sighted; young [Greek]

D

Dacian	From the place name, Dacia
Dacre	From the surname; from Dacre, Cumbria; trickling stream [Celtic]
Dacso	Hungarian form of Daniel; God is my judge [Hebrew]
Daemon	Variant of Damian; to tame [Greek]
Daeron	Variant of Darren, a variant of Darrell
Daffydd	Welsh variant of David; beloved [Hebrew]
Dag	From the Norse god's name; daylight [Old Norse]
Dagget	Elaborate form of Dag; from the Norse God's name; daylight [Old Norse]
Dakota	Friends [Dakota/Native American]
Dale	From the surname; person living in a dale/valley

Daley From the surname; assembly [Gaelic]
Dallas From the surname; from Dallas, Scotland; meadow dwelling. Or for Dallas, Texas
Dalton From the surname; from the valley town [Old English]
Daly Variant of Daley; from the surname; assembly [Gaelic]

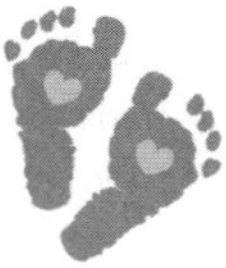

Damian To tame [Greek]
Damien Variant of Damian; to tame [Greek]
Damon Variant of Damian; to tame [Greek]
Dan Diminutive of Daniel; God is my judge [Hebrew]
Dana From the surname; Dane; from Denmark
Dane Variant of Dean; from the surname; from the valley; or working as or for a dean
Daniel God is my judge [Hebrew]
Dannie Diminutive of Daniel; God is my judge [Hebrew]
Danny Diminutive of Daniel; God is my judge [Hebrew]
Darby From the surname; from the town of Derby; deer [Old Norse]
Darcy From the surname; coming from town of Arcy, France
Darell Variant of Darrell; from the surname; coming from Airelle. France [Norman French]
Daren Form of Darren, a variant of Darrell; coming from Airelle. France [Norman French]
Darian Form of Darren, variant of Darrell; coming from Airelle. France [Norman French]
Darien Form of Darren, a variant of Darrell; coming from Airelle. France [Norman French]
Darin Form of Darren, a variant of Darrell; coming from Airelle. France [Norman French]
Darion Form of Darren, a variant of Darrell; coming from Airelle. France [Norman French]
Darius Possesses good [Persian]
Darnell From the surname; from the hidden nook [Old English]
Darrel Variant of Darrell; from the surname; coming from Airelle. France [Norman French]
Darren Variant of Darrell; from the surname; coming from Airelle. France [Norman French]
Darrin Variant of Darren, a variant of Darrell; coming from Airelle. France [Norman French]
Darryl Variant of Darrell; from the surname; coming from Airelle. France [Norman French]
Darwin From the surname; dear friend [Old English]
Daryl Variant of Darrell; from the surname; coming from Airelle. France [Norman French]
Dashiell English form of the French surname de Chiel
Dave Diminutive of David; beloved [Hebrew]
Davey Diminutive of David; beloved [Hebrew]
David Beloved [Hebrew]
Davie Diminutive of David; beloved [Hebrew]
Davin Variant of Devin; from the surname; fawn [Gaelic]; or from the English county Devon
Davis From the surname, derived from David; beloved [Hebrew]
Davy Diminutive of David; beloved [Hebrew]
Dawson From the surname; son of David; beloved [Hebrew]
Dax From the surname; from Dax, France
Daxton Invented name; elaborate form of Dax
Dayton From the surname; from the dairy town, or ditch town [Old English]
Deacon Deacon, cleric [Greek].
Dean From the surname; from the valley; or working as or for a dean
Declan Man of prayer

Dee	Diminutive of names beginning with D-. Or for the River Dee in Scotland
Deforest	From the surname; from the forest
Delano	From a French surname; from La Noue; from the swamp [French]
Delbert	Diminutive of Adalbert, a variant of Albert; noble one; bright [Old German]
Dell	One who lives in a dell/valley. Or diminutive of Derek
Delmar	From the surname, de la mare; from the sea, lake, pond [Norman French]
Delroy	Variant of Leroy; the king [French]. Or Dell + Roy
Den	Diminutive of Dennis; god from Nysa [Greek]
Dene	Variant of Dean; from the surname; from the valley; or working as or for a dean
Denholm	From the surname; from the valley island [Old English]
Denis	Variant of Dennis; god from Nysa [Greek]
Dennis	Form of Dionysius; god from Nysa [Greek]
Denny	Diminutive of Dennis; god from Nysa [Greek]
Denton	From the surname; from the valley town [Old English]
Denver	From the valley ford [Old English]. Or for the US city Denver, Colorado
Denzel	Variant of Denzil; from a surname; from Denzell, Cornwall
Denzil	From a surname; from Denzell, Cornwall.
Deon	Variant of Dion; god [Greek]
Derby	From the surname; from the town of Derby; deer [Old Norse]
Derek	Variant of Theodoric; ruler of the people [Greek]
Derick	Variant of Derek; ruler of the people [Greek]
Deren	Variant of Darren, variant of Darrell; coming from Airelle. France [Norman French]
Derrick	Variant of Derek; ruler of the people [Greek]
Derryl	Variant of Darrell; coming from Airelle. France [Norman French]
Deryck	Variant of Derek; ruler of the people [Greek]
Des	Diminutive of Desmond; from the Irish surname; from South Munster [Irish]
Desmond	From the Irish surname; from South Munster [Irish]
Devan	Variant of Devin; fawn [Gaelic]; or from the English county Devon
Deven	Variant of Devin; fawn [Gaelic]; or from the English county Devon
Devereux	From the surname; from Evreux, France [French]
Devin	From the surname; fawn [Gaelic]; or from the English county Devon
Devon	From the English county Devon. Or variant of Devin; fawn [Gaelic]
Devyn	Variant of Devin; fawn [Gaelic]; or from the English county Devon
Dewayne	Variant of Duane; from an Irish surname; small, dark one [Irish]
Dex	Diminutive of Dexter; from the surname; dyer [Old English]. Or skilled [Latin]
Dexter	From the surname; dyer [Old English]. Or right-handed, skilled [Latin]
Dexy	Diminutive of Dexter; from the surname; dyer [Old English]. Or skilled [Latin]
Dezi	Diminutive of Desmond; from the Irish surname; from South Munster [Irish].
Dick	Diminutive of Richard; brave, powerful one [Old German]
Digby	From the town of Digby; farm by the ditch [Old English/Old Norse]
Diggory	Lost one [Old French]
Dillan	Variant of Dylan; great one from the sea [Welsh]
Dillon	Variant of Dylan; great one from the sea [Welsh]. Or loyal [Irish]
Dion	God [Greek]

Dirk	Diminutive of Diederik/Theodoric; ruler of the people [Greek]. Or Scottish dagger
Dixon	From the surname; son of Dick; brave, powerful one [Old German]
Dolph	Diminutive of Adolph; noble wolf [Old German]
Dom	Diminutive of Dominic; of the Lord [Latin]
Domenic	Variant of Dominic; of the Lord [Latin]
Dominic	Of the Lord [Latin]
Dominick	Variant of Dominic; of the Lord [Latin]
Don	Diminutive of Donald; ruler of the world [Gaelic]
Donald	Ruler of the world [Gaelic]
Donnie	Diminutive of Donald; ruler of the world [Gaelic]
Donny	Diminutive of Donald; ruler of the world [Gaelic]
Donovan	From the Irish surname; small, dark brown one [Gaelic]
Dorian	Invented by Oscar Wilde. From the Ancient Greek tribe, Dorians. Wanderer [Gaelic]
Doug	Diminutive of Douglas; from the Scottish surname; dark river [Gaelic]
Dougie	Diminutive of Douglas; from the Scottish surname; dark river [Gaelic]
Douglas	From the Scottish surname; dark river [Gaelic]
Drake	From the surname; dragon [Old Norse & Old English]
Dre	Diminutive of Andre; variant of Andrew, from the French André; strong [Greek]
Drew	Diminutive of Andrew; strong; manly [Greek]
Driscoll	From the Irish surname; messenger [Irish]
Driskoll	Variant of Driscoll; from the Irish surname; messenger [Irish]
Drogo	One who carries; ghost; precious [Old German/Norman]
Drummond	From the Scottish surname; from the ridge [Gaelic]
Duane	From an Irish surname; small, dark one [Irish]
Dudley	From the surname; from Dudda's clearing [Old English]
Duke	From the noble title or the surname; leader [Latin]
Duncan	Brown warrior [Gaelic]
Dunstan	Dark stone [Old English]
Durward	From the surname; door guard [Old English]
Dustin	Thor's stone [Old Norse]
Dusty	From a nickname; dusty. Or diminutive of Dustin; Thor's stone [Old Norse]
Dutch	From an American nickname given to people of German descent
Dwain	Variant of Duane; from an Irish surname; small, dark one [Irish]
Dwayne	Variant of Duane; from an Irish surname; small, dark one [Irish]
Dwight	From the surname; a feminine variant of of Dion; god [Greek]
Dylan	Great one from the sea [Welsh]
Dyson	Son of Dye, a medieval diminutive of Dionisia; god from Nysa [Greek]

E

Eamon	Irish form of Edmund; wealthy protector
Earl	From the noble title; nobleman; warrior [Old English/Norse]
Earle	Variant of Earl; from the noble title; nobleman; warrior [Old English/Norse]
Earnest	Variant of Ernest; serious [Old German]
Easton	From the surname; from the east town [Old English]
Eben	Diminutive of Ebenezer; helpful stone; stone of help [Hebrew]
Ebenezer	Helpful stone; tone of help [Hebrew]
Ed	Diminutive of Edward, Edmund and other names beginnin with Ed-
Eddie	Diminutive of Edward, Edmund and other names beginnin with Ed-
Eddy	Diminutive of Edward, Edmund and other names beginnin with Ed-
Eden	From the Biblical garden; place of pleasure [Hebrew]
Edgar	Wealthy spearsman [Old English]
Edison	Son of Eda/Edith; spoils of war [Old English]. Or son of Adam; man [Hebrew]
Edmund	Wealthy protector [Old English]
Edric	Wealthy ruler [Old English]
Edward	Wealthy guard [Old English]
Edwin	Wealthy friend [Old English]
Edwyn	Variant of Edwin; welathy friend [Old English]
Egan	Variant of Aidan; little fore [Irish]
Egbert	Bright sword-edge; bright blade [Old English]
Eldon	From the surname; from Ella's hill [Old English]
Eldred	From the surname; old cousellor [Old English]
Eleazer	Variant of Lazarus; God is my helper [Hebrew]
Elgar	Spearman [Old English]
Eli	Ascension [Hebrew]
Elias	Variant of Elijah; my God is Jehova [Hebrew]
Elijah	My God is Jehova [Hebrew]
Eliot	Variant of Elliott; from a surname derived from Elijah; my God is Jehova [Hebrew]
Eliott	Variant of Elliott; from a surname derived from Elijah; my God is Jehova [Hebrew]
Ellery	Masculine form of Hilary; cheerful [Latin/Greek]
Elliot	Variant of Elliott; from a surname derived from Elijah; my God is Jehova [Hebrew]
Elliott	From a surname derived from Elijah; my God is Jehova [Hebrew]
Ellis	Variant of Elliott; from a surname derived from Elijah; my God is Jehova [Hebrew]
Ellison	Son of Ellis; from a surname derived from Elijah; my God is Jehova [Hebrew]
Elmer	From the surname; noble and famous [Old English]
Elmo	Protection; protector [Old German]

Elroy Variant of Leroy; the king [French]
Elsdon From the surname; from Elli's valley [Old English]
Elton From the surname; from Ella's town [Old English}
Elvin Variant of Alvin; elf friend [Old English}
Elvis Unknown meaning; possibly a variant of Alvis; all wise [Old Norse]
Elwin Variant of Alvin; elf friend [Old English}
Elwood From the surname; from the elder tree forest [Old English]
Elwyn Variant of Alvin; elf friend [Old English}
Ely Variant of Eli; ascension [Hebrew]
Emerson From the surname; son of Emery; universal power [Old German]
Emery Universal power [Old German]
Emil From a Roman family name; rival [Latin]
Emlen Variant of Emil/Emlyn; rival [Latin]
Emlyn Welsh variant of Emil; rival [Latin]
Emmanuel God is with us [Hebrew]
Emmet Variant of Emmett; a diminutive of Emma; whole; universal [Old German]
Emmett From the surname; a diminutive of Emma; whole; universal [Old German]
Emory Variant of Emery; universal power [Old German]
Ennis Variant of Angus; one strength [Gaelic]
Enoch Dedicated [Hebrew]
Enrique Spanish form of Henry; home ruler [Old German]
Enrico Italian variant of Henry; home ruler [Old German]. Diminutive of Vincenzo, Lorenzo
Enys Variant of Enys/Angus; one strength [Gaelic]
Eoin Irish variant of Owen; well-born [Greek; youth [Welsh]. Or Irish form of John
Erastus Beloved [Greek]
Eric Always ruler [Old Norse]
Erick Variant of Eric; always ruler [Old Norse]
Erik Variant of Eric; always ruler [Old Norse]
Erle Variant of Earl; from the noble title; nobleman; warrior [Old English/Norse]
Ern Diminutive of Ernest; serious [Old German]
Ernest Serious [Old German]
Ernie Diminutive of Ernest; serious [Old German]
Erny Diminutive of Ernest; serious [Old German]
Errol From a surname; from Errol, Scotland;
Erskine From the surname; from Erskine, Scotland; projecting height [Gaelic]
Esme Variant of Esmé; esteemed; loved [Old French]
Esmé Esteemed; loved [Old French]
Esmond Grace; protection [Old English]
Esmund Variant of Esmons; grace; protection [Old English]
Esteban Spanish form of Stephen; crown; honour; reward [Greek]
Estefan Variant of Esteban; Spanish form of Stephen; crown; honour; reward [Greek]
Ethan Firm; enduring [Hebrew]
Ethelbert Old English variant of Albert; noble; bright
Ethelred Noble cousellor [Old English]

Eugene Well-born [Greek]
Eustace Fruitful [Greek]
Evan Anglicized variant of Iefan, Welsh form of John; God is gracious [Hebrew]
Evander Anglicized form of Iomhar, a Scottish form of Ivor; yew bow warrior [Old Norse]
Evelyn From the surname; desired [Old German]
Everard Brave boar {Old German]
Everett Variant of Everard; brave boar [Old German]
Everette Variant of Everard; brave boar [Old German]
Everitt Variant of Everard; brave boar [Old German]
Ewart From the surname, derived from Edward; wealthy guard [Old English]
Ezekiel God strenghens [Hebrew]
Ezra Help [Hebrew]

F

Faber Variant of Fabian; bean-grower [Latin]
Fabian Bean-grower [Latin]
Fabiano Elaborate form of Fabio/Fabian; bean-grower [Latin]
Fabio Bean-grpwer [Latin]
Fabron Young blacksmith [French]
Faraday From the surname; wood man [Gaelic]
Farley From the surname; from the fern clearing [Old English]
Faron From a French surname; from Faro
Farran From the surname; iron grey [Old French]
Farrell From the surname; Anglicized form of Fearghal; man of valour [Gaelic]
Fearghal Man of valour [Gaelic]
Feargus Variant of Fergus; man of vigour [Gaelic]
Felipe Spanisjh form of Philip; friend of horses [Greek]
Felix Lucky; successful [Latin]
Fennel From the plant
Fenton From the surname; from the marsh town [Old English]
Feodor Russian form of Theodore; gift of God [Greek]
Ferdie Diminutive of Ferdinand; brave journey [Old German]
Ferdinand Brave journey; brave voyager [Old German]
Ferdy Diminutive of Ferdinand; brave journey [Old German]
Fergie Diminutive of Fergus; man of vigour [Gaelic]
Fergus Man of vigour [Gaelic]
Fernando Spanish variant of Ferdinand; brave voyager [Old German]
Field Field; or from the surname

Fielder	From the surname; field dweller; one who lives in open country [Old English]
Fielding	From the surname; one who lives or works in fields/open country [Old English]
Filbert	Brilliant [Old German]
Fin	Variant of Finn; fair; white [Gaelic]
Finbar	Fair-haired [Irish]
Findlay	Variant of Finlay; fair warrior [Gaelic]
Fineas	Variant of Phineas; oracle [Hebrew]
Finlay	Fair warrior [Gaelic]
Finley	Variant of Finlay [Gaelic]
Finn	Fair; white [Gaelic]
Finnegan	From the Irish surname; small, fair one {Gaelic]
Fisher	From the surname; one who fishes
Fisk	From the surname; fisherman [Old English]
Fitz	Prefix denoting illegitimate son of, e.g. Fitzroy; son of the king [Norman French]
Fitzroy	(Illegitimate) son of the king {Norman French]
Flanagan	From the Irish surname; small, red-haired one [Gaelic]
Flannery	From the Irish surname; red valour [Gaelic]
Fletcher	From the surname; arrow maker [Old French]
Florian	Flowering [Latin]
Florin	Flower; flourishing [Latin]
Floyd	From the surname; variant of Lloyd; grey [Welsh]
Flynn	From the surname; red; red-haired one [Irish]
Ford	From the surname; living near a ford
Forest	Forest. Or from the surname; living/working in a forest
Forrest	Variant of Forest; forest. Or from the surname; living/working in a forest
Fort	Strong [Latin/French]
Fortney	Strong one [Latin]
Fortune	Luck; wealth [Latin]
Fortuno	Spanish variant of Fortune; luck; wealth [Latin]
Foster	Variant of Forester; forest worker. Or scissor maker, wood worker [Old French]
Fox	From the surname; for the animal. Or from a nickname.
Fran	Diminutive of Francis; French/Frankish man
Francesco	Italian form of Francis; French/Framnkish man
Francis	French/Frankish man
Francisco	Spanish & Portuguese form of Francis; French/Frankish man
Frank	Diminutive of Francis; French/Frankish man
Frankie	Diminutive of Francis; French/Frankish man
Franklin	From the surname; free man [Old English]
Franklyn	Variant of Franklin; from the surname; free man [Old English]
Franny	Diminutive of Francis; French/Frankish man
Fraser	Scottish surname; from strawberry place [French]; curly-haired; or forest men
Frasier	Scottish surname; from strawberry place [French]; curly-haired; or forest men
Frazer	Scottish surname; from strawberry place [French]; curly-haired; or forest men
Frazier	Variant of Fraser; from strawberry place [French]; curly-haired; or forest men

Fred Diminutive of Frederick; peaceful ruler [Old German]
Freddie Diminutive of Frederick; peaceful ruler [Old German]
Freddy Diminutive of Frederick; peaceful ruler [Old German]
Frederick Peaceful ruler [Old German]
Fredric Variant of Frederick; peaceful ruler [Old German]
Fredrick Variant of Frederick; peaceful ruler [Old German]
Freedman From the surname; one who has been freed
Freeland From the surname; from the free land. Or variation of Freeman
Freeman From the surname; free man
French From the surname or country name; from France
Frey Lord; exalted one [Old Norse]
Frisco Diminutive of Francisco; French/Frankish man. Or ickname for San Francisco
Friso Frisian; from Friesland, Netherlands
Fritz Diminutive of Frederick; peaceful ruler [Old German]
Frost From the surname or weather condition; frost; frosty-haired
Fulk People [Old German]
Fulke Variant of Fulk; people [Old German]
Fulton From the surname; from the town of Foulden, Norfolk; bird hill [Old English]
Fynn Variant of Finn; fair; white [Gaelic]
Fyodor Russian form of Theodore; gift of God [Greek]

G

Gabby Diminutive of Gabriel; God is my strength [Hebrew]
Gabe Diminutive of Gabriel; God is my strength [Hebrew]
Gable From the surname; gable; side end of a building
Gabriel God is my strength [Hebrew]
Gabo Diminutive of Gabriel; God is my strength [Hebrew]
Gabor Hungarian form of Gabriel; God is my strength [Hebrew]
Gad Diminutive of Gadiel; God is my fortune [Arabic/Hebrew]
Gadge Variant of Gage; measurer, assayer; or moneylender [Old French]
Gadiel God is my fortune [Arabic/Hebrew]
Gaelan Variant of Galen; calm [Greek]
Gaetan From Gaeta [Italian/Latin]
Gage From the surname; measurer, assayer; or moneylender [Old French]
Gaines From the surname; employer of trickery [Old English]
Gale From the surname; jovial [Old English]
Galen Calm [Greek]
Galo From Gaul [Latin]

Gallagher From the Irish surname; stranger help [Irish]
Galloway From the Scottish surname; foreigner; stranger [Gaelic]
Galt High ground [Old Norse]
Galton From the surname; from a rented estate [Old English]
Galvin Sparrow [Irish]
Gannon From the surname; fair colouring [Irish]
Gareth Gentleness [Welsh]
Garey Variant of Gary; spear [Old German].
Garfield From the surname; from or owning a triangular field [Old English]
Garland From the surname; owning triangular shaped land [Old English]
Garnet Hinge maker [Old French]. Or French Guarin; guard; protector [Old German]
Garnett Hinge maker [Old French]. Or French Guarin; guard; protector [Old German]
Garret Variant of Garrett; rule of the spear. Or from Gerard; hardy spear [Old German]
Garrett From the surname; rule of the spear. Or from Gerard; hardy spear [Old German]
Garrick From the surname; from the grove of oak trees [Occitan French]
Garry Variant of Gary; spear [Old German].
Garth From the surname; garden/gardener; one who lives near a garden [Old Norse]
Gary Spear; spear bearer [Old German]
Gaspar Spanish variant of Casper/Jasper; treasurer [Persian]
Gaspard French variant of Casper/Jasper; treasurer [Persian]
Gaston Foreigner; guest [Old German]
Gates From the surname; one living near city gates
Gatsby From the surname; left-handed; from Gat [Old German]
Gauge Variant of Gage; from the surname; measurer, assayer; or moneylender [Old French]
Gauguin From the French surname
Gauthier French form of Walter; ruler of the army [Old German]
Gauvan Variant of Gavin/Gawain; hawk of May [Welsh]
Gavan Variant of Gavin/Gawain; hawk of May [Welsh]
Gaven Variant of Gavin/Gawain; hawk of May [Welsh]
Gavin Variant of Gawain; hawk of May [Welsh]

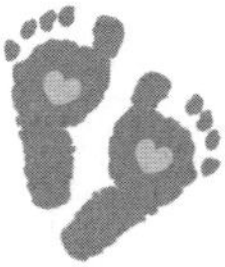

Gavril Arabic and East European variant of Gabriel; God is my strength [Hebrew]
Gavyn Variant of Gawain/Gavin; hawk of May [Welsh]
Gaz Diminutive of Gary; spear [Old German]. Or of Gareth; gentleness [Welsh]
Geffrey Variant of Geoffrey; hostage of peace [Old German]
Gene Diminutive of Eugene; well born [Greek]
Genet Eden [African]
Genio Italian & Spanish diminutive of Eugene; well-born [Greek]
Gennaro January [Italian/Latin]
Geno Italian & Spanish diminutive of Eugene; well-born [Greek]
Geoff Diminutive of Geoffrey; hostage of peace [Old German]
Geoffrey Hostage of peace [Old German]
Geordie Diminutive of George; farmer [Greek]
George Farmer [Greek]
Georgie Diminutive of George; farmer [Greek]

Gerald Rule of the spear [Old German]
Gerard Hardy spear [Old German]
Germain French form of Germanus; brother [Latin]
German English form of Germanus; brother [Latin]
Gerome Variant of Jerome; sacred name [Greek]
Geronte Variant of Gareth; gentleness [Welsh]
Gerrald Variant of Gerald; rule of the spear [Old German]
Gerrard Variant of Gerard; hardy spear [Old German]
Gerell Variant of Gerald; rule of the spear [Old German]
Gerrick Variant of Garrick; from the grove of oak trees [Occitan French]
Gerrit Variant of Gerard; hardy spear [Old German]
Gerry Diminutive of Gerald; rule fo the spear, Or of Gerard; hardy spear [Old German]
Gervase Servant spear [Old German]
Gib Diminutive of Gilbert; bright pledge [Old German]
Gideon Hewer; feller; warrior [Hebrew]
Giffard From the surname; brave; gift [Old German]
Gil Diminutive of Gilbert; bright pledge [Old German]
Gilad Variant of Gilead; from the Biblical place name; camel hump [Hebrew]
Gilam Variant of Gili; my joy [Hebrew]
Gilbert Bright pledge [Old German]
Gilead From the Biblical place name; camel hump [Hebrew]
Gilean Variant of Giles; young goat [Greek]
Giles Young goat [Greek]
Gili My joy [Hebrew]
Gino Italian diminutive of Eugene; well born [Greek]
Gio Diminutive of Giovanni, Italian form of John; God is gracious {Hebrew]
Giotto Italian form of Godfrey; peace of God; hostage/pledge of peace [Hebrew]
Giovanni Italian form of John; God is gracious {Hebrew]
Gladwin From the surname; bright friend [Old English]
Gladwyn Variant of Gladwin; from the surname; bright friend [Old English]
Glanville From the surname; from Glan's domain [Norman French]
Glen Variant of Glenn; from the Scottish surname; from the glen/valley [Gaelic]
Glenn From the Scottish surname; from the glen/valley [Gaelic]
Glenwood From the surname; from the wooded glen/valley
Glin Variant of Glenn; from the Scottish surname; from the glen/valley [Gaelic]
Glover From the surname; one who makes/sells gloves
Glynn Welsh form of Glenn; from the valley/glen
Goddard From the surname; good and brave; bravery of God [Old German]
Godfrey Peace of God [Old German]
Goodwin From the surname; friend of God [Old German]
Gord Diminutive of Gordon; from the Scottish surname; of the spacious fort
Gordie Diminutive of Gordon; from the Scottish surname; of the spacious fort
Gordon From the Scottish surname; of the spacious fort
Gordy Diminutive of Gordon; from the Scottish surname; of the spacious fort

Gore	From the surname; from a triangular piece of land [Old English]
Gosse	From the surname; a Norman form of Gozzo; little Goth [Old German]
Grady	From the Irish surname; noble [Gaelic]
Graeme	From the Scottish surname; variant of Graham; gravelly home [Old English]
Graham	From the Scottish surname; from Grantham; gravelly home [Old English]
Grahame	From the Scottish surname; variant of Graham; gravelly home [Old English]
Gram	Diminutive of Graham; from the Scottish surname; gravelly home [Old English]
Gramercy	From the name of a Manhattan park, New York
Grange	Variaqnt of Granger; from the surname; granary worker [Old English]
Granger	From the surname; granary worker [Old English]
Granite	From the name of the hard stone
Grant	From the surname; great [Norman French]
Grantley	Variant of Grant; from the surname; great [Norman French]
Granville	From the surname; from Grainville, Guarin's town [Norman French]
Gray	From the surname; one with grey hair/grey clothing
Grayson	From the surname; son of the steward [Old English]
Greer	From a Scottish surname related to Gregor; watchful {Greek]
Greg	Diminutive of Gregor and Gregory; watchful [Greek]
Gregg	Diminutive of Gregor and Gregory; watchful [Greek]
Gregor	Variant of Gregory; watchful [Greek]
Gregory	Watchful [Greek]
Grenville	Variant of Granville; from the surname; from Grainville, Guarin's town [French]
Gresham	From the surname; from the "grazing homestead" [Old English]
Grey	Variant of Gray; from the surname; one with grey hair/grey clothing
Greyson	Variant of Grayson; from the surname; son of the steward [Old English]
Grier	Variant of Greer; from a Scottish surname related to Gregor; watchful {Greek]
Griffin	Latinized form of Gruffudd; strong lord/prince [Welsh]
Griffith	Strong lord/prince [Welsh]
Grigor	Variant of Gregor/Gregory; watchful [Greek]
Grosvenor	From theh surname; great hunter [Norman French]
Grover	From the surname; from the grove [Old English]
Gruff	Gruff
Gryffon	Variant of Griffin; strong lord/prince [Welsh]
Gualtiero	Italian form of Walter; ruler of the army [Old German]
Gunner	Scandinavian variant of Gunther; bold warrior [Old German/Norse]
Gunther	Bold warrior [Old German]
Gus	Diminutive of Augustus; great [Latin]. Or of Angus; one strength [Gaelic]
Gustaf	Variant of Gustav; staff or rod of the Goths [Old German]
Gustav	Staff or rod of the Goths [Old German]
Gustavo	Latin variant of Gustav; staff or rod of the Goths [Old German]
Guthrey	Variant of Guthrie; from the Scottish surname. Scotland; from a windy place [Gaelic]
Guthrie	From the Scottish surname; from Guthrie, Scotland; from a windy place [Gaelic]
Guy	Norman French form of Wido; wood; wide [Old German]
Gwylym	Welsh form of Willian; resolute protector [Old German]

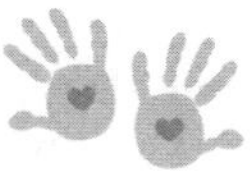

Gyan	Full of knowledge [Sanskrit]
Gyle	Variant of Giles; young goat [Greek]. Or path through a bog [Scots]
Gyles	Variant of Giles; young goat [Greek]
Gyon	Dutch form of Guy, Norman French form of Wido; wood; wide [Old German]

H

Haakon	Chosen son [Old Norse]
Habib	Loved one [Arabic]
Haco	Flame; fire [Celtic]
Hackett	From the surname; little hewer [Old German]
Hadar	Splendour; citrus fruit [Hebrew]
Hadaram	Elaborate form of Hadar; splendour; citrus fruit [Hebrew]
Haden	Variant of Hayden; from the surname; from the hay valley or hay hill [Old English]
Hadley	From the surname; from the heather field [Old English]
Hadrian	Dark-haired [Latin]
Hadriel	Splendour of God [Hebrew]
Hadyn	Variant of Hayden; from the surname; from the hay valley or hay hill [Old English]
Hagen	Variant of Haakon; chosen son [Old Norse]
Haig	From the surname; from a place enclosed with hedges [Old English/Armenian]
Hale	From the surname; one who lives in a hollow [Old English]
Hainey	Varaint of Haines; from the surname; from the cottage with vines [Old German]
Haines	From the surname; from the cottage with vines [Old German]
Haji	Born during the pilgrimage to Mecca [Swahili]
Hakan	Fiery [Native American]
Hal	Medieval diminutive of Harry/Henry; home ruler [Old German]
Hale	From the surname; from the nook or retreat [Old English]
Hall	From the surname; one who lives or works in a great hall/manor house
Hallam	From the surname; one who lives at the rocks; or at the nook [Old English]
Ham	Hot; warm [Hebrew]
Hamid	Variant of Muhammed; praised one; praiseworthy [Arabic]
Hamilton	From the surname; from the crooked hill [OldEnglish]
Hamish	Scottish form of James; supplanter [Hebrew]
Hamlin	Little home lover [Old German]
Hammond	From the surname; home protection [Old German]; high protection [Old Norse]
Hamnet	Diminutive of Hamo; home [Old German]
Hampton	From the surname; from Hampton; from the home settlement [Old English]
Hamza	Lion [Arabic]
Handley	Variant of Henley; from the surname; from the high meadow [Old English]

Hank Diminutive of John; God is gracious [Hebrew]. Home ruler [Old German

Hannibal Grace of Baal [Assyrian & Punic]

Happy Happy

Harald Variant of Harold; army ruler [Old English & Old Norse]

Harding From the surname; hardy [Old English]

Hardy From the surname; hardy [Old English]

Harlan From the surname; land of hare [Old English]

Harland Variant of Harlan; from the surname; land of hare [Old English]

Harley From the surname; from the hare wood clearing [Old English]

Harlow From the surname; from the rock hill; from the army hill [Old English]

Harmon From the surname; variant of Herman; army man [Old German]

Harold Army ruler [Old English & Old Norse]

Harper From the surname; one who plays or makes the harp

Harpo From the nickname

Harrald Variant of Harold; army ruler [Old English & Old Norse]

Harrell God's mountain [Hebrew]

Harrington From the surname; from the family farm; one who works around the manor house

Harris From the surname; derived from Harry, diminutive of Henry; home ruler [German]

Harrison From the surname; son of Harry, diminutive of Henry; home ruler [Old German]

Harro Diminutive of Heinrich/Henry; home ruler [Old German]

Harrold Variant of Harold; army ruler [Old English & Old Norse]

Harry Diminutive of Henry; home ruler [Old German]

Hart From the name of the animal; stag

Harte Variant of Harte; from the name of the animal; stag. Or from the surname

Hartley From the surname; from the hart clearing [Old English]

Harve Diminutive of Harvey; battle worthy [Breton]

Harvey Battle worthy [Breton]

Harvie Variant of Harvey; battle worthy [Breton]

Haven Haven; safe place [Old English]

Hayden From the surname; from the hay valley or hay hill [Old English]

Haydn From the German surname; heathen [Old German]

Hayes From the surname; from the hedged land [Old English]

Hayward Protector of the hedge enclosure [Old English]

Haywood From the surname; from the enclosed wood [Old English]

Haze Variant of Hayes; from the surname; from the hedged land [Old English]

Hazen Variant of Hayes; from the surname; from the hedged land [Old English]

Headley Variant of Hedley; from the surname; from the heather clearing [Old English]

Heath From the surname; one who lives on the heath [Old English]

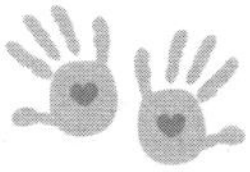

Hector Possess; hold fast [Greek]

Hedley From the surname; from the heather clearing [Old English]

Heller From the surname; bright; brilliant [Old German]

Hemingway From the surname; from the place name [English]

Henderson From the Scottish surname; son of Henry; home ruler [Old German]

Hendrie From the Scottish surname; son of Henry; home ruler [Old German]

Hendrix	From Hendrick, Scandinavian and Dutch form of Henry; home ruler [Old German]
Henley	From the surname; from the high meadow [Old English]
Henning	Danish form of Henry; home ruler [Old German]
Henry	Home ruler [Old German]
Herb	Diminutive of Herbert; army bright [Old German]
Herbert	Army bright [Old German]
Herbie	Diminutive of Herbert; army bright [Old German]
Herman	Army man [Old German]
Hershel	Deer [Hebrew]
Hervey	Variant of Harvey; battle worthy [Breton]
Hew	Variant of Hugh; spirit; heart [Old German]
Hewett	From the surname; French diminutive of Hugh; spirit; heart [Old German]
Hewie	Variant of Hughie, diminutive of Hugh; spirit; heart [Old German]
Hewson	From the surname; variant of Houston; from Houston; Hugh's town
Hilary	English form of Hilarius; cheerful [Latin/Greek]
Hildred	Battle counsellor [Old English]
Hiram	Exalted brother [Hebrew]
Hobart	Variant of Hubert; bright heart [Old German]
Hobie	Diminutive of Hobart, a variant of Hubert; bright heart [Old German]
Hobey	Diminutive of Hobart, a variant of Hubert; bright heart [Old German]
Hogan	Youth [Irish]
Hoke	From the surname
Holden	From the surname; from the deep valley [Old English]
Hollis	From the English surname; one who lives by the holly trees [Old English]
Homer	Hostage; pledge [Greek]
Hooper	From the surname; one who makes hoops
Horace	English form of Roman family name Horatius; of the time, season, hour [Latin]
Horatio	English form of Roman family name Horatius; of the time, season, hour [Latin]
Horst	Leap [Old German]
Horton	From the surname; from the grey settlement [Old English]
Hoseah	Salvation [Hebrew]
Houston	From the Scottish surname; from Houston; Hugh's town
Howard	Brave heart [Old German]; high guardian [Old Norse]; or ewe herder [Old English]
Howe	From the surname; from the hill [Old German]
Howel	From the surname; from the hilly land [Old English]
Howie	Brave heart [Old German]; high guardian [Old Norse]; or ewe herder [Old English]
Hoy	From the surname; sailor on a cargo ship [Old German/Dutch]
Hoyt	From the surname; stick; one who is stick thin [Old English]
Hubert	Bright heart [Old German]
Hubbell	Brave heart [Old German]
Hubble	Variant of Hubbell; brave heart [ld German]
Huck	Diminutive of Huckleberry; from the name of the fruit/plant
Huckleberry	From the name of the fruit/plant
Hudson	Son of Hudde, a diminutive of Hugh; heart; spirit [Old German]

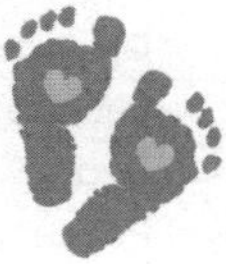

Huey	Diminutive of Hugh; heart; spirit [Old German]
Hugh	Heart; spirit [Old German]
Hughie	Diminutive of Hugh; heart; spirit [Old German]
Hugo	Latinized form of Hugh; heart; spirit [Old German]
Humbert	Bright warrior [Old German]
Humphrey	Peaceful warrior [Old German]
Humphry	Variant of Humphrey; peaceful warrior [Old German]
Hunter	From the surname; hunter
Hyde	From the surname; from Hyde; from a unit of land. Or to hide
Hyram	Variant of Hiram; exalted brother [Hebrew]
Hyrum	Variant of Hiram; exalted brother [Hebrew]
Hywell	Welsh variant of Howel; from the surname; from the hilly land

I

Iagan	Scottish form of Egan; little fire [Gaelic]
Iago	Welsh form of James/Jacob; supplanter [Hebrew]
Ian	Scottish form of John; God is gracious [Hebrew]
Iain	Variant of Ian, Scottish form of John; God is gracious [Hebrew]
Ibo	My people [African]
Ibrahim	Arabic variant of Abraham; father of multitudes [Hebrew]
Ibsen	From the surname; son of Ib, diminutive of Jacob/James; supplanter [Hebrew]
Idris	Lord [Welsh]
Iggy	Diminutive of Ignatius; from a Roman family name, later associated with fire
Ilya	Russian form of Elias/Elijah; my God is Jehova [Hebrew]
Ignatius	From a Roman family name; fire; burbing; ardent
Ike	Diminutive of Isaac; he will laugh; he will rejoice [Hebrew]
Iker	Visitation [Basque]
Ilario	Cheerful; happy [Greek]
Ilarion	Variant of Ilario; cheerful; happy [Greek]
Ilbert	From the English surname derived from Hildbert; battle bright [Old German]
Indiana	From the name of the US state; land of the Indians
Indigo	From the colour [Greek]
Inglis	From the surname; variant of Ingram; raven of the Angles [Old German]
Ingmar	Son of Ing [Old Norse]
Ingram	From the surname; Angle raven; raven of the Angles [Old German]
Inigo	My little love [Basque]. Also associated with Ignatius
Innes	From the Scottish surname; from the river island [Gaelic]
Innis	Variant of Innes; from the Scottish surname; from the river island [Gaelic]

Ira	Watchful [Hebrew]
Irvin	From the surname; variant of Irving; from the place of green water
Irvine	Variant of Irving; from the Scottish surname; from the place of green water
Irving	From the Scottish surname; from the place of green water
Irwin	From the surname; boar friend [Old English]
Isaac	He will laugh; he will rejoice [Hebrew]
Isador	Variant of Isidore; gift of Isis [Greek/Egyptian]
Isadore	Variant of Isidore; gift of Isis [Greek/Egyptian]
Isaiah	God is salvation [Hebew]
Isiah	Variant of Isaiah; God is salvation [Hebew]
Isidore	Gift of Isis [Greek/Egyptian]
Israel	God contended [Hebrew]
Issac	Variant of Isaac; he will laugh; he will rejoice [Hebrew]
Issy	Diminutive of Isidore and other names beginning with Is-
Ivan	Slavic form of John; God is gracious [Hebrew]
Ivo	Variant of Ivor; bow warrior; yew warrior [Old Norse]
Ivor	Bow warrior; yew warrior [Old Norse]
Izzy	Diminutive of Isidore, and other names beginning with Is-

J

Jabari	Comforter; consoler [Swahili]
Jabe	Diminutive of Jabez; borne in pain [Hebrew]
Jabez	Borne in pain [Hebrew]
Jac	Variant of Jack, a diminutive of John; God is gracious [Hebrew]
Jace	Diminutive of Jason; to heal; healer [Greek]
Jack	Diminutive of John; God is gracious [Hebrew]
Jackie	Diminutive of Jack/John; God is gracious [Hebrew]
Jackson	From the surname; son of Jack, a diminutive of John; God is gracious [Hebrew]
Jacob	Holder of the heel; supplanter [Hebrew]
Jacobi	Variant of Jacob; supplanter [Hebrew]
Jacoby	Variant of Jacob; supplanter [Hebrew]
Jacot	Variant of Jacques, French form of James/Jacob; supplanter [Hebrew]
Jacques	French form of James/Jacob; supplanter [Hebrew]
Jaden	God has heard; judge; thankful [Hebrew]
Jadyn	Variant of Jaden; God has heard; judge; thankful [Hebrew]
Jae	Variant of Jay; diminutive of names beginning with J-
Jaiden	Variant of Jaden; God has heard; judge; thankful [Hebrew]
Jalen	James + Leonard

Jake	Medieval variant of Jack, diminutive of John. Or of Jacob; supplanter [Hebrew]
Jamal	Beauty [Arabic]
Jamar	Variant of Jamal; beauty [Arabic]
James	English form of Jacob; supplanter [Hebrew]
Jameson	From the surname; son of James; supplanter [Hebrew]
Jamey	Diminutive of James, English form of Jacob; supplanter [Hebrew]
Jamie	Diminutive of James, English form of Jacob; supplanter [Hebrew]
Jamison	From the English surname; son of James; supplanter [Hebrew]
Jan	Variant of John; God is gracious [Hebrew]
Janek	Polish variant of John; God is gracious [Hebrew]
Janus	Gateway [Greek]
Jared	Descent [Hebrew]
Jarod	Variant of Jared; descent [Hebrew]
Jaron	Jared + Darren
Jarred	Variant of Jared; descent [Hebrew]
Jarrett	Variant of Garrett; derived from Gerald; rule of the spear, hardy spear [Old German]
Jarrod	Variant of Jared; descent [Hebrew]
Jarvis	From the surname; derived from Gervais; servant spear [Old German]
Jason	To heal; healer [Greek]
Jasper	Treasurer [Persian]
Javan	Greece [Hebrew]
Jaxon	Variant of Jackson; son of Jack, a diminutive of John; God is gracious [Hebrew]
Jaxson	Variant of Jackson; son of Jack, a diminutive of John; God is gracious [Hebrew]
Jay	Diminutive of names beginning with J-
Jayce	Diminutive of Jason; to heal; healer [Greek]
Jaycob	Variant of Jacob; supplanter [Hebrew]
Jayden	Variant of Jaden; God has heard; judge; thankful [Hebrew]
Jaydon	Variant of Jaden; God has heard; judge; thankful [Hebrew]
Jaylen	Variant of Jalen; James + Leonard
Jaylin	Variant of Jalen; James + Leonard
Jaymes	Variant of James; supplanter [Hebrew]
Jayson	Variant of Jason; to heal; healer [Hebrew]
Jazz	From the musical genre. Or diminutive of Jasper; treasurer [Persian]
Jeb	Diominutive of Jacob; supplanter [Hebrew]
Jed	Diminutive of Jedidiah; beloved of God [Hebrew]
Jedidiah	Beloved of God [Hebrew]
Jeff	Short form of Jeffrey, variant of Geoffrey; hostage of peace [Old German]
Jefferson	From thesurname; son of Jeffrey/Geoffrey; hostage of peace [Old German]
Jeffery	Variant of Geoffrey; hostage of peace [Old German]
Jeffrey	Variant of Geoffrey; hostage of peace [Old German]
Jeffry	Variant of Geoffrey; hostage of peace [Old German]
Jem	Diminutive of Jeremy; God has lifted [Hebrew]. Or of James; supplanter [Hebrew]
Jemmy	Diminutive of Jeremy; God has lifted [Hebrew]. Or of James; supplanter [Hebrew]
Jenson	Son of Jens, a Scandinavian form of John; God is gracious [Hebrew]

Jep	Diminutive of Geoffrey; hostage of peace [Old German]
Jepson	Son of Jep, a diminutive of Geoffrey; hostage of peace [Old German]
Jephthah	He opens [Hebrew]
Jeptha	Variant of Jephthah; he opens [Hebrew]
Jerald	Variant of Gerald; rule of the spear [Old German]
Jere	Diminutive of Jeremiah; God has lifted [Hebrew]
Jeremiah	God has lifted [Hebrew]
Jeremy	English form of Jeremiah; God has lifted [Hebrew]
Jermaine	Variant of Germane; French form of Germanus; brother [Latin]
Jerold	Variant of Gerald; rule of the spear [Old German]
Jerome	Sacred name [Greek]
Jerrard	Variant of Gerard; hardy spear [Old German]
Jerred	Variant of Jared; descent [Hebrew]
Jerrod	Variant of Jared; descent [Hebrew]
Jerrold	Variant of Gerald; rule of the spear [Old German]
Jerry	Diminutive of Jeremy, Gerald etc.
Jervis	From the surname; variant of Jarvis/Gervais; servant spear [Old German]
Jess	Short form of Jesse; gift [Hebrew
Jesse	Gift [Hebrew]
Jessie	Variant of Jesse; gift [Hebrew]
Jesus	The Lord is salvation [Hebrew]
Jethro	Excellence [Hebrew]
Jett	From the precious stone; black; or from the aircraft
Jevon	Welsh form of Evan/John; God is gracious [Hebrew]
Jewel	Precious stone. Or from the surname; generous prince [Old Breton]
Jewell	Variant of Jewel; precious stone. Generous prince [Old Breton]
Jez	Diminutive of Jeremy; God has lifted [Hebrew]. Or of James; supplanter [Hebrew]
Jezza	Diminutive of Jeremy; God has lifted [Hebrew]. Or of James; supplanter [Hebrew]
Jim	Diminutive of James; supplanter [Hebrew]
Jimi	Diminutive of James; supplanter [Hebrew]
Jimmie	Diminutive of James; supplanter [Hebrew]
Jimmy	Diminutive of James; supplanter [Hebrew]
Jiro	Second son [Japanese]
Jo	Diminutive of Joseph, Jonathan and other names beginning with Jo-
Job	Persecuted; hated [Hebrew]
Joby	Diminutive of Job; persecuted; hated [Hebrew]
Jocelyn	From Gaul [Old German]
Jody	Diminutive of Joseph; he will add [Hebrew]
Joffrey	Scottish variant of Jeffrey/Geoffrey; hostage of peace [Old German]
Joe	Diminutive of Joseph; he will add [Hebrew]
Joel	Jehova is God {Hebrew]
Joey	Diminutive of Joseph; he will add [Hebrew]
Johan	German form of John; God is gracious [Hebrew]
John	God is gracious [Hebrew]

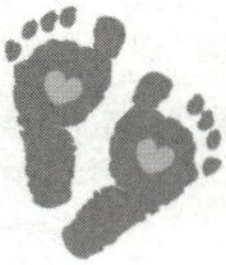

Johnathan	Variant of Jonathan; God has given [Hebrew]
Johnathon	Variant of Jonathan; God has given [Hebrew]
Johnie	Diminutive of John; God is gracious [Hebrew]
Johnnie	Diminutive of John; God is gracious [Hebrew]
Johnny	Diminutive of John; God is gracious [Hebrew]
Johnson	From the surname; son of John; God is gracious [Hebrew]
Jojo	Diminutive of Joseph, Jonathan and other names beginning with Jo-
Jolyon	Variant of Julian; downy-bearded [Latin]
Jon	Diminutive of Jonathan; God has given [Hebrew]. Or variant of John]
Jonah	Dove [Hebrew]
Jonathan	God has given [Hebrew]
Jonathon	Variant of Jonathan; God has given [Hebrew]
Jones	From the surname; derived from John; God is gracious [Hebrew]
Jonny	Variant of Jonathan; God has given [Hebrew]
Jonson	Variant of Johnson; from the surname; son of John; God is gracious [Hebrew]
Jonty	Diminutive of Jonathan; God has given [Hebrew]
Jools	Diminutive of Julian; downy-bearded [Latin]
Jordan	From the name of the river
Jordon	Variant of Jordan; from the name of the river
Jos	Diminutive of Joseph; he will add [Hebrew]
Jose	Spanish & Portuguese form of Joseph; he will add [Hebrew]
Josef	Variant of Joseph; he will add [Hebrew]
Joseph	He will add [Hebrew]
Josh	Diminutive of Joshua; God is salvation [Hebrew]
Joshua	God is salvation [Hebrew]
Josiah	God supports [Hebrew]
Joss	Diminutive of Jocelyn; from Gaul [Old German]
Jovan	Majestic; love [Latin]. Or Slavic form of John; God is gracious; [Hebrew]
Joyce	Lord [Old Breton]
Judd	Diminutive of Jordan; from the name of the river
Judas	Prasied {Hebrew]
Jude	Variant of Judas; praised [Hebrew]
Jules	Diminutive of Julian; downy-bearded [Latin]
Julian	From the Roman name Iulianus/Julius; downy-bearded [Latin]
Julio	Spanish form of Julius; downy-bearded [Latin]
Julius	From the Roman family name; downy-bearded [Latin]
Julyan	Variant of Julian; downy-bearded [Latin]
Junior	From a nickname for a boy name after his father
Justice	From the surname; judge, justice
Justin	Just [Latin]
Justy	Diminutive of Justin; just

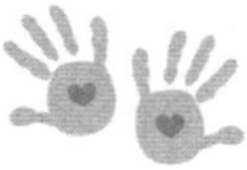

K

Kade	Variant of Cade; from the surname derived from a nickname; round [Old English]
Kaden	Variant of Caden; spirit of battle [Gaelic]. Or friend; companion [Arabic]
Kadir	Capable [Arabic]
Kaeden	Variant of Caden; spirit of battle [Gaelic]. Or friend; companion [Arabic]
Kafka	From the surname; jackdaw [Czech]
Kahil	Variant of Kahlil; friend [Arabic]
Kai	Sea [Hawaian]
Kaiden	Variant of Caden; spirit of battle [Gaelic]. Or friend; companion [Arabic]
Kain	Variant of Cain; acquired; possessed [Hebrew]
Kaleb	English variant of Caleb; dog; whole heart [Hebrew]
Kam	Diminutive of Cameron; from the Scottish surname; crooked nose [Gaelic]
Kamal	Lotus; perfection [Hindi/Arabic]
Kameron	Diminutive of Cameron; from the Scottish surname; crooked nose [Gaelic]
Kano	God of the waters [African/Japanese]
Kanye	From the Nigerian place name; honour; tribute [African]
Kaolin	Anglicized form of Caolan; small, slender one [Gaelic]
Karl	German & Scandinavian form of Charles; warrior [Old German]
Kasey	Variant of Casey; from the surname; vigilant [Irish]
Kasimir	German variant of Casimir; destroyer of fame/prestige; proclaims peace [Slavic]
Kason	Invented name to rhyme with Cason, Jason, Mason etc
Kaspar	Scandinavian form of Caspar; treasurer [Persian]
Kavan	Battle [Breton]
Kayden	Variant of Caden; spirit of battle [Gaelic]. Or friend; companion [Arabic]
Keane	English form of Cian; from the surname; ancient [Gaelic]
Keaton	From the surname; from the shed town [Old English]
Keefe	From the Irish surname; kind, handsome, gentle [Gaelic]
Keegan	From the Irish surname; son of fire; little fire [Gaelic]
Keene	Variant of Kean; from the surname; English form of Cian; ancient [Gaelic]
Keenon	From the surname; Irish diminutive of Cian; ancient [Gaelic]
Kees	Dutch diminutive of Cornelius; from the Roman family name; of the horn [Latin]
Kegan	Variant of Keegan; from the Irish surname; son of fire; little fire [Gaelic]
Keir	From the surname; variant of Kerr; from rough, wet ground [Old Norse]
Keiran	Variant of Kieran/Ciaran; little, dark one [Gaelic]
Keith	From the Scottish surname; from Keith; from the wood [Celtic]
Kelcey	Variant of Kelsey; from the surname; from Cenel's island [Old English]
Kellan	Swamp; slender [German/Irish]
Kellen	Variant of Kellan; swamp; slender [German/Irish]

Kelley	Variant of Kelly; from the surname; bright-headed; war; church [Irish]
Kelly	From the surname; bright-headed; war; church [Irish]
Kelsey	From the surname; from Cenel's island [Old English]
Kelso	From the Scottish surname and place name
Kelton	From the surname; from the town of the keels [Old English]
Kelvan	Variant of Kelvin; from the Scottish river; narrow water
Kelvin	From the Scottish river; narrow water
Kemal	Variant of Kamal; lotus; perfection [Hindi/Arabic]
Kemp	From the surname; champion; warrior [Old English]
Ken	Diminutive of Kenneth; handsome; born in fire [Gaelic]
Kendal	From the surname; variant of Kendall; from Kendale; from the valley of the river Kent
Kendall	From the surname; from Kendale; from the valley of the river Kent
Kendrick	Royal power; bold power [Old English]; chief hero [Welsh]; son of Henry [Gaelic]
Kenelm	Keen protection [Old English]
Kenith	Variant of Kenneth; handsome; born in fire [Gaelic]
Kennard	From the surname; royal guard [Old English]
Kennedy	From the Irish surname; armoured head [Gaelic]
Kenneth	Handsome; born in fire [Gaelic]
Kennett	Scandinavian form of Kenneth; handsome; born in fire [Gaelic]
Kennith	Variant of Kenneth; handsome; born in fire [Gaelic]
Kenny	Diminutive of Kenneth; handsome; born in fire [Gaelic]
Kenrick	Royal power; bold power [Old English]; chief hero [Welsh]; son of Henry [Gaelic]
Kent	From the surname; from Kent, England; coastal district [Celtic]
Kenton	From the surname; town on the River Kenn; from the royal town [Old English]
Kenyon	From the surname; from a place name; unknown meaning
Kenzie	Contraction of MacKenzie; from the surname; handsome [Gaelic]
Kermit	From the Manx surname; son of Diarmaid; without envy [Irish]
Kern	Variant of Ciaran; little dark person [Gaelic]
Kerr	From the Scottish surname; from rough, wet ground [Old Norse]
Kerrigan	From the surname; from County Kerry, Ireland; Ciar's people
Kerry	From the name of the Irish county; Ciar's people
Kester	Scottish form of Christopher; bearing Christ; carrying Christ [Greek]
Kev	Diminutive of Kevin; gentle birth [Irish]
Keveen	Variant of Kevin; gentle birth [Irish]
Kevin	Gentle birth [Irish]
Kevyn	Variant of Kevin; gentle birth [Irish]
Kian	Variant of Cian; acient [Gaelic]
Kiaran	Anglicized form of Ciaran; little dark person, little person with black hair [Gaelic]
Kiefer	From a German surname; from near the pine tree; or barrel maker [Old German]
Kier	From rough, wet ground [Old Norse]. Diminutive of Kieran; small, dark one [Gaelic]
Kieth	Variant of Keith; from the Scottish surname; from Keith; from the wood [Celtic]
Kilan	Diminutive of Kyle; from the kyle; narrows, channel [Gaelic]
Killian	Variant of Cillian; little church; little strife [Irish]
Kim	Diminutive of Kimberley, from the South African city. Or of Kimball; war chief; bold

Kimball	War chief [Welsh]; bold [Old English]
King	From a nickname; king; kingly [Old English]
Kingsley	From the surname; from the king's wood [Old English]
Kingston	From the surname; from Kingston; king's town [Old English]
Kip	From kipper; male salmon in spawning season; one who smokes/cures fish
Kipling	From the surname; from Cybbel's cottage [Old English]
Kirby	From the surname; from Kirby; church settlement [Old Norse]
Kirk	From the surname; church [Old Norse]
Kit	Diminutive of Christopher; bearing Christ; carrying Christ [Greek]
Knox	From the Scottish surname; from the round hill [Old English]
Koby	Variant of Coby; diminutive of Jacob; supplanter [Hebrew]
Kodey	Variant of Cody; from the surname; helpful [Irish]
Kody	Variant of Cody; from the surname; helpful [Irish]
Kofi	Born on Friday [Twi]
Kolby	Variant of Colby; from the surname; dark town; coal town [Old Norse]
Kole	Variant of Cole; charcoal; one who is dark-featured [Old English]
Kolin	Variant of Colin; dove [Latin]. Diminutive of Nicholas; victory of the people [Greek]
Konnor	Variant of Conor; dog-lover; wolf-lover [Gaelic]
Korbin	Variant of Corbin; from the surname; raven; one with black hair [French]
Korey	Variant of Corey; from the surname; hollow-dweller; spear
Kory	Variant of Corey; from the surname; hollow-dweller; spear
Kris	Variant of Chris; short form of Kristian, Kristopher.
Kristopher	Variant of Christopher; bearing Christ; carrying Christ [Greek]
Kurt	Brave counsellor [Old German]. Or diminutive of Curtis; courteous [Old French]
Kurtis	Variant of Curtis; courteous [Old French]
Kyle	From the Scottish surname; from the kyle; narrows, channel [Gaelic]
Kyler	Variant of Kyle. Scottish: from the kyle; narrows, channel [Gaelic].
Kynaston	From the surname; from Cynefrid's town; royal peace [Old English]
Kyra	Throne [Persian]
Kyrie	Variant of Kyra; throne [Persian]; lord [Greek]

L

Laban	White [Hebrew]
Labe	Diminutive of Laban; white [Hebrew]
Lacey	From the surname; variant of Lacy; from Lassy, Normandy
Lachlan	From Norway; from land of lochs/fjords; from far away [Gaelic]
Lachlann	Variant of Lachlan; from Norway; from land of lochs/fjords; from far away [Gaelic]
Lacy	From the surname; from Lassy, Normandy

Ladislas Variant of Vladislav; glorious ruler [Slavic]
Ladislav Variant of Vladislav; glorious ruler [Slavic]
Lael Belonging to God [Hebrew]
Lafayette Faith [French]
Lago Spanish form of Lake; lake; living near a lake
Laird From a Scottish surname; lord; landowner
Lake Lake; living near a lake [Latin]
Lamar From the surname; from the water, pool, sea [Norman French]
Lambert From the surname; from the bright land [Old German]
Lamont From the Scottish surname; law man [Old Norse]
Lampard Variant ofLambert; from the surname; from the bright land [Old German]
Lance Possessor of land; lance; spear [Old German]
Landen Variant of Landon; from the surname; from the long hill [Old English]
Lando Diminutive of names ending in -lando
Landon From the surname; from the long hill [Old English]
Lane From the surname; from the lane or path [Old English]
Lanford From the surname; from the long ford [Old English]
Langdon Variant of Landon; from the surname; from the long hill [Old English]
Langston From the surname; long stone [Old English]
Lanny Diminutive of names beginning with Lan-
Larrie Diminutive of Laurence; from the Roman name; from Laurentum [Latin]
Larry Diminutive of Laurence; from the Roman name; from Laurentum [Latin]
Lars Scandinavian form of Laurence; from the Roman name; from Laurentum [Latin]
Laszlo Glorious ruler [Hungarian]
Lauren French variant of Laurence; from the Roman name; from Laurentum [Latin]
Laurence From the Roman name Laurentius; from Laurentum [Latin]
Laurie Diminutive of Laurence; from the Roman name; from Laurentum [Latin]
Lavern Variant of Laverne; from the surname; from the place of alder trees [French]
Laverne From the surname; from the place of alder trees [French]
Lawrence Variant of Laurence; from the Roman family name; from Laurentum [Latin]
Lawrie Diminutive of Lawrence/Laurence; from the Roman name; from Laurentum [Latin]
Lawson From the surname; son of Laurence; from Laurentum [Latin]
Layne Variant of Lane; from the surname; from the lane or path [Old English]
Layton From the surname; from the town/village with a leek garden [Old English]
Laz Diminutive of Laurence; from the Roman name; from Laurentum [Latin]
Lazarus God is my helper [Hebrew]
Lebron The brown-haired one [French]
Lebrun Variant of Lebron; the brown-haired one [French]
Lech Pole; Polish person [Polish]
Ledger From the surname; the people's spear [Old German]
Lee From the surname; from the clearing [Old English]
Legend Legend
Leigh From the surname; variant of Lee; from the clearing [Old English]
Leighton Variant of Layton; from the town/village with a leek garden [Old English]

Leith	From the surname; from Leith, near Edinburgh; wet, damp. From the Water of Leith
Leland	From the surname; from the fallow land [Old English]
Lemoine	From a French surname; the monk [French]
Lemond	Variant of Lamont; from the Scottish surname; law man [Old Norse]
Lemuel	Devoted to God [Hebrew]
Len	Diminutive of Leonard; brave lion [Old German]
Lenard	Variant of Leonard; brave lion [Old German]
Lennard	Variant of Leonard; brave lion [Old German]
Lennie	Diminutive of Leonard; brave lion [Old German]
Lennon	From the Irish surname; lover [Gaelic]
Lennox	From the Scottish surname; from Lennox, place of elms [Gaelic]
Lenny	Diminutive of Leonard; brave lion [Old German]
Lenox	From the surname; variant of Lennox; from Lennox, place of elms [Gaelic]
Leo	Lion [Latin]
Leon	Lion [Greek]
Leonard	Brave lion [Old German]
Leopold	Bold people [Old German]
Leroi	Variant of Leroy; the king [Old French]
Leroy	French nickname; the king [Old French]
Les	Diminutive of Leslie; holly garden. Or of Lester; from the surname; from Leicester
Lesley	Variant of Leslie; from the Scottish surname; from Leslie; holly garden [Gaelic]
Leslie	From the Scottish surname; from Leslie; holly garden [Gaelic]
Lester	From the surname; from the city of Leicester
Levi	Joined [Hebrew]
Lewin	From the surname; dear friend [Old English]
Lewis	English form of Louis; famous in battle [Old German]
Lex	Diminutive of Alexander; the defender [Greek]
Leyland	Variant of Leland; from the surname; from the fallow land [Old English]
Leyton	Variant of Layton; from the town/village with a leek garden [Old English]
Liam	Irish diminutive of William; resolute protector [Old German]
Light	Light
Lilburn	From the surname; from the village of Lilburn or Lilbourne
Lincoln	From Lincoln; from the settlement by the lake, pool [Celtic/Latin]
Linden	From the surname; lime tree [German]
Lindon	From the surname; variant of Lyndon; from the lime tree hill [Old English]
Lindsay	From the surname; from Lindsay, Lincolnshire
Lindsey	Variant of Lindsay; from the surname; from Lindsay, Lincolnshire
Lindy	Diminutive of Lindbergh; possibly from the dance, the Lindy Hop
Linford	From the surname; from the flax ford; or from the lime tree ford [Old English]
Linton	From the surname; from the flax ford; or from the lime tree ford [Old English]
Linus	Flax [Greek]
Linwood	From the surname; from the forest stream [Old English]
Lio	Variant of Leo; lion [Latin]
Lionel	French diminutive of Leon; lion [Greek]

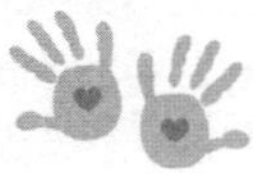

Lir	From the sea [Irish]
Litton	From the surname; from the hill settlement [Old English]
Llewellyn	Leader's choice [Welsh]
Lloyd	From the surname; grey [Welsh]
Llyr	From the sea [Welsh]
Loch	Loch; lake [Gaelic]
Lochlan	Variant of Lachlan; from Norway; from land of lochs/fjords; from far away [Gaelic]
Lochlin	Variant of Lachlan; from Norway; from land of lochs/fjords; from far away [Gaelic]
Lochran	From the surname; rushes [Irish]
Logan	From the Scottish surname; from the little hollow [Gaelic]
Loman	From the surname; delicate [Irish]
Lon	Diminutive of names containing -lon-
Lonan	Blackbird [Irish]
London	London, United Kingdom
Lonnie	Diminutive of names containing -lon-
Lonny	Diminutive of names containing -lon-
Loren	Diminutive of Laurence; from the Roman family name; from Laurentum [Latin]
Lorin	Diminutive of Laurence; from the Roman family name; from Laurentum [Latin]
Lorn	Variant of Lorne; from Lorne, Scotland
Lorne	From Lorne, Scotland
Lorrin	Diminutive of Laurence; from the Roman family name; from Laurentum [Latin]
Lou	Diminutive of Louis; famous in battle [Old German]
Loudon	From the surname; from the low valley [Old German]
Louie	Diminutive of Louis; famous in battle [Old German]
Louis	Famous in battle [Old German]
Lovel	From the surname; variant of Lowell; little wolf [Norman French]
Lovell	From the surname; variant of Lowell; little wolf [Norman French]
Lowell	From the surname; little wolf [Norman French]
Loyal	Loyal; faithful
Loyd	Variant of Lloyd; From the surname; grey [Welsh]
Luc	Variant of Luke; from Lucania, southern Italy [Greek]
Luca	Italian variant of Luke; from Lucania, southern Italy [Greek]
Lucas	Variant of Luke; from Lucania, southern Italy [Greek]
Lucian	English form of Roman family name Lucianus; light [Latin]
Lucifer	Light bearer [Latin]
Lucius	Light [Latin]
Lucky	Lucky; or diminutive of Luke; from Luciana, southern Italy [Greek]
Lude	Diminutive of Ludovic, English form of Louis; famous in battle [Old German]
Ludek	Czech variant of Louis/Ludovic; famous in battle [Old German]
Ludlow	From the surname; from the ruler's hill [Old English]
Ludo	Diminutive of Ludovic, English form of Louis; famous in battle [Old German]
Ludovic	English form of Louis; famous in battle [Old German]
Ludwig	German form of Louis; famous in battle [Old German]
Luis	Variant of Louis; famous in battle [Old German]

Luiz Spanish form of Louis; famous in battle [Old German]
Luke From Lucania, southern Italy [Greek]
Luther my people; famous warrior [Old German]. Or lute player [Old English]
Lyall From the Scottish surname; wolf [Old Norse]
Lyle From the surname; from the island [Norman French]
Lyndon From the surname; from the lime tree hill [Old English]
Lynn From the surname; lake [Welsh]
Lynton Variant of Linton; from the flax ford; or from the lime tree ford [Old English]
Lynwood Variant of Linwood; from the surname; from the forest stream [Old English]
Lysander Liberator [Greek]
Lytton Variant of Litton; from the surname; from the hill settlement [Old English]

M

Macaire French form of Makari; blessed [Greek]
Macallister From the Scottish surname; son of Allister/Alexander; the defender [Greek]
Macaulay From the Scottish surname; son of the righteous [Gaelic]
Mack From the surname; diminutive of surnames beginning with Mac/Mc; son of [Gaelic]
Mackenzie From the surname; son of the handsome one [Gaelic]
Maclean From the Scottish surname; servant of St. John [Gaelic
Maddox From the Welsh surname; son of Madoc; fortunate little one [Welsh]
Maddison Variant of Madison; from the surname; son of Maud
Madison From the surname; son of Maud
Mael Lord; chief; prince [Celtic]
Maes From the Dutch surname; son of Thomas; twin [Aramaic]
Magnus Greatest [Latin]
Maitland From the surname; from the inhospitable place [Norman French]
Major From the surname; council spear [Old German]. Or major; important; significant
Makari Blessed [Greek]
Malachi My messenger; my angel [Hebrew]
Malakai Variant of Malachi; my messenger; my angel [Hebrew]
Malcolm Follower of Sant Columba [Gaelic]
Malcom Variant of Malcolm; follower of Sant Columba [Gaelic]
Malek Variant of Malik; king [Arabic]
Malick Variant of Malik; king [Arabic]
Malik King [Arabic]
Maliq Variant of Malik; king [Arabic]
Malo Shining hostage [Breton]
Malone From the Irish surname; follower of Saint John [Irish]

Mandela	From the African surname; circle; symbol of the universe [Sanskrit]
Manley	From the surname; from the common clearing [Old English]
Manny	Diminutive of Emmanuel; God is with us [Hebrew]
Mansel	From the surname; from the French city of Le Mans
Manuel	Spanish& Portuguese form of Emmanuel; God is with us [Hebrew]
Marcello	Young warrior [Latin]
Marcus	Of the Roman god, Mars; warrior [Latin]
Maria	Sometimes masculine middle name; sea of sorrow; wished for child [Hebrew]
Marino	Of the sea [Latin]
Mario	Variant of Marius; name of the Roman god, Mars; warrior [Latin]
Marion	Diminutive of Mary/Marie/Maria; sea of sorrow; bitter; wished for child [Hebrew]
Marius	From the Roman family name; of the Roman god, Mars; warrior [Latin]
Mark	Form of Marcus; of the Roman god, Mars; warrior [Latin]
Marley	From the surname; from a seaside meadow [Old English]
Marlin	Variant of Merlin; sea fortress [Welsh]
Marlon	Meaning uncertain; perhaps little falcon
Marlowe	From the surname; from Marlowe; remnants of a lake [Old English]
Marmaduke	English variant of Mael Maedoc; followe of Saint Maedoc [Welsh]
Marsden	From the surname; from the boundary valley [Old English]
Marshal	Variant of Marshall; from the surname; marshal [Old German]
Marshall	From the surname; marshal [Old German]
Martie	Diminutive of Martin; of the Roman god, Mars [Latin]
Martin	Of the Roman god, Mars [Latin]
Marty	Diminutive of Martin; of the Roman god, Mars [Latin]
Marvin	Variant of Mervyn; marrow famous [Welsh]
Marvyn	Variant of Marvin/Mervyn; marrow famous [Welsh]
Maso	Italian diminutive of Thomas; twin [Aramaic]
Mason	From the surname; stoneworker [Old German]
Massimo	Italian variant of Maximus; the greatest [Latin]
Masterman	From the surname; one who worked as a servant.
Mat	Diminutive of Matthew; gift of God [Hebrew]
Matai	Variant of Matthew; gift of God [Hebrew]
Mateo	Sapanish form of Matthew; git of God [Henrew
Mathew	Variant of Matthew; gift of God [Hebrew]
Matt	Diminutive of Matthew; gift of God [Hebrew]
Matteo	Italian form of Matthew; gift of God [Hebrew]
Matthew	Gift of God [Hebrew]
Matthias	Variant of Matthew; gift of God [Hebrew]
Mattie	Diminutive of Matthew; gift of God [Hebrew]
Matty	Diminutive of Matthew; gift of God [Hebrew]
Maurice	From the Roman name, Mauritius/Marius; dark-skinned [Latin]
Maverick	Maverick; independent
Max	Form of Maximilian; greatest [Latin]..Magnus's stream [Old English/Norse]
Maximilian	Greatest [Latin]

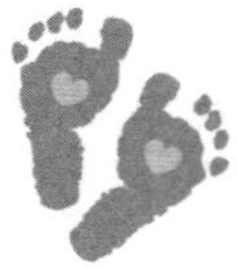

Maximillian Variant of Maximilian; greatest [Latin]

Maxwell From the Scottish surname; from Mack's/Magnus's stream [Old English/Norse]

Maynard From the surname; hardy strength [Old German]

Maynerd Variant of Maynard; from the surname; hardy strength [Old German]

Mayson Variant of Mason; from the surname; stoneworker [Old German]

Meade One who lived on a meadow; maker or seller of mead [Old English]

Mel Diminutive of names beginning with Mel-

Melville From the Scottish surname; from the bad town [Norman French]

Melvin From the Scottish surname; from the bad town [Norman French]

Melvyn Variant of Melvin; from the bad town [Norman French]

Memphis Enduring and beautiful [Greek]

Meredith Great lord; sea lord [Welsh]

Merit Variant of Merritt; the boundary gate [Old English]. Or merit; deserving [Latin]

Meriwether From the surname; happy weather; cheerful person

Merle Variant of Merrill; bright sea [Bretan]

Merlin Sea fortress [Welsh]

Merlyn Variant of Merlin; sea fortress [Welsh]

Merrick Derived from Meurig, Welsh form of Maurice; dark-skinned [Latin]

Merrill From the surname, derived from Muriel; bright sea [Gaelic]

Merritt From the surname; from the boundary gate [Old English]

Merton From the surname; from the town on a lake [Old English]

Merv Diminutive of Mervyn; marrow famous [Welsh]

Mervin Variant of Mervyn; marrow famous [Welsh]

Mervyn Marrow famous [Welsh]

Messiah Deliverer; expected saviour [Aramaic]

Meurig Welsh form of Maurice; from the Roman name, Mauritius; dark-skinned [Latin]

Meyer Bringer of light; Hebrew.

Micah Contracted form of Micaiah; who is like God? [Hebrew]

Michael Who is like God? [Hebrew]

Micheal Variant of Michael; who is like God? [Hebrew]

Mick Diminutive of Michael; who is like God? [Hebrew]

Mickey Diminutive of Michael; who is like God? [Hebrew]

Micky Diminutive of Michael; who is like God? [Hebrew]

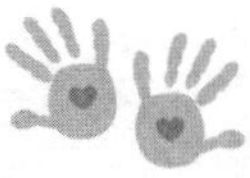

Miguel Spanish form of Michael; who is like God? [Hebrew

Mike Diminutive of Michael; who is like God? [Hebrew]

Mikey Diminutive of Michael; who is like God? [Hebrew]

Mikhail Russian form of Michael; who is likle God? [Hebrew]

Milburn From the surname; from the mill stream [Old English]

Miles Variant of Milo; gracious [Slavic]; or soldier [Latin]

Milford From the surname; from the ford by a mill [Old English]

Millard From the surname; guardian of the mill [Old English]

Miller From the surname; miller; grinder of grain

Milo Gracious [Slavic]; or soldier [Latin]

Milton From the surname; from the mill town" [Old English]

Miro	Peace; world [Slavic]
Mitch	Short form of Mitchell; derived from Michael; who is like God? {Hebrew]
Mitchell	From the surname, derived from Michael; who is like God? {Hebrew]
Mo	Diminutive of names beginning with the sound Mo-
Moe	Diminutive of names beginning with the sound Mo-
Monroe	From the Scottish surname; from the mouth of the River Roe
Montague	From the surname; pointed mountain [Old French]
Montana	From the name of the US state; mountainous [Latin]
Monte	Diminutive of Montgomery; from Gumarich's mountain [Norman French]
Montgomery	From the surname; from Gumarich's mountain [Norman French]
Monty	Variant of Monte; from Gumarich's mountain [Norman French]
Mordecai	Servant of Marduk, a Babylonian god [Persian]
Mordikai	Variant of Mordecai; servant of Marduk, a Babylonian god [Persian]
Morgan	Sea defender [Welsh]
Morley	From the surname; from the marsh clearing [Old English]
Morris	Variant of Maurice; from the Roman name, Mauritius/Marius; dark-skinned [Latin]
Mort	From the moor town [Old English]. From the still water; dead water [Old French]
Mortimer	From the surname; from the still water; dead water [Old French]
Morton	From the surname; from the moor town [Old English]
Morty	From the moor town [Old English]. From the still water; dead water [Old French]
Moses	Son [Egyptian]; deliver [Hebrew]
Moss	Medieval form of Moses; son [Egyptian]; deliver [Hebrew]
Muhammad	Turkish variant of Muhammed; praised one; praiseworthy [Arabic]
Muhammed	Praised one; praiseworthy [Arabic]
Murphy	From the Irish surname; sea warrior [Irish]
Murray	From the Scottish surname; from Moray, seaboard settlement
Myles	Variant of Miles; gracious [Slavic]; or soldier [Latin]
Myron	Sweet oil; perfume [Greek]

N

Nabil	High born [Arabic]
Nachman	Variant of Nachum; comforter [Hebrew]
Nachum	Comforter [Hebrew]
Nadim	Friend; drinking companion [Arabic]
Nagel	From the German surname; nail maker [Old German]
Naim	River with alder trees [Gaelic]
Nairn	From the name of the Scottish town; river with alder trees [Gaelic]
Nando	Diminutive of Fernando; brave voyager [Old German]

Napier	From the surname; linen keeper [Old French]
Napoleon	Sons of mist [Corsican/Old German]; or lion of Naples [Latin]
Nardo	Diminutive of Bernardo/Bernard; strong as a bear [Old German]
Nash	From the surname; at the ash tree [Old English]
Nasser	Winner [Arabic]
Nat	Diminutive of Nathan; he gave [Hebrew]. Or of Nathaniel; God has given [Hebrew]
Nate	Diminutive of Nathan; he gave [Hebrew]. Or of Nathaniel; God has given [Hebrew]
Nathan	He gave [Hebrew]
Nathaniel	God has given [Hebrew]
Nathon	Variant of Nathan; he gave [Hebrew]
Naveed	Good news [Persian]
Naylor	From the surname; nailer; carpenter
Neal	Variant of Neil/Niall; chaampion; or cloud [Gaelic]
Ned	Diminutive of Edward; wealthy guard, wealthy protector [Old English]
Neely	From the Scottish surname; son of the poet [Gaelic]
Neil	Variant of Niall; champion; or cloud [Gaelic]
Nelson	From the surname; son of Neil; son of the champion; or cloud [Gaelic]
Nerio	Variant of Nerius; water; sea [Greek]
Nerius	Water; sea [Greek]
Nero	Stern [Latin]
Nevil	Variant of Neville; from the surname; from the new town [Norman French]
Neville	From the surname; from the new town [Norman French]
Newt	Diminutive of Newton; from the surname; from the new town [Old English]
Newton	From the surname; from the new town [Old English]
Nic	Diminutive of Nicholas; victory of the people [Greek]. Or of Dominic; of the Lord
Nicholas	Victory of the people [Greek]
Nick	Diminutive of Nicholas; victory of the people [Greek]
Nickolas	Variant of Nicholas; victory of the people [Greek]
Nicky	Diminutive of Nicholas; victory of the people [Greek]
Nico	Diminutive of Nicholas; victory of the people [Greek]
Nicol	Variant of Nicholas; victory of the people [Greek]
Nicolas	Variant of Nicholas; victory of the people [Greek]
Nigel	Latin form of Neil; champion; cloud [Gaelic]; also influenced niger, black [Latin]
Nigellus	Latin form of Nigel/Neil; champion; cloud [Gaelic];
Nik	Diminutive of Nicholas; victory of the people [Greek]
Nikolai	Russian form of Nicholas; victory of the people [Greek]
Nikolas	Variant of Nicholas; victory of the people [Greek]
Nile	Variant of Niall/Neil; champion; or cloud [Gaelic]. From the name of the river Nile
Niles	From the surname, derived from Neil/Niall; champion; or cloud [Gaelic]
Nils	Norwegian form of Nicholas; victory of the people [Greek]
Nilsson	From the Scandinavian surname; son of Nils; victory of the people [Greek]
Ninian	Meaning unknown, from the saint's name.
Noah	Rest; comfort [Hebrew]
Noble	From the surname; noble; notable; aristocratic

Noel	English form of Noël; Christmas [French]
Nolan	From the Irish surname; noble or famous little one [Irish]
Norbert	North bright [Old German]
Norm	Diminutive of Norman; northman; Viking [Old German]
Norman	Northman; Viking [Old German]
Normand	From the surname; Norman; Viking [Old Germna]
Norris	From the north [Old French]. Or foster mother/wet nurse [Old French]
Norton	From the surname; from the north town [Old English]
Norville	From the surname; from a northern town [Old English/French]
Norwood	From the surname; from the north wood [Old English]
Nowell	From the surname; variant of Noel; Christmas
Nygel	Variant of Nigel, Latin form of Neil; champion; cloud [Gaelic]

O

Oak	From the name of the tree
Oakes	From the surname; one who lives near the oak trees
Oakley	From the surname; from the oak wood or clearing [Old English]
Obadiah	Servant of God [Hebrew]
Obama	Leaning; bending; flexible [Luo]. Or surname, place name; little beach [Japanese]
Oberon	Noble; bear like [Old German]
Ocean	Ocean; sea
Octavian	Eighth; eighth child or child born in the eighth month [Latin]
Odell	From the surname; from the woad hill [Old English]
Odilio	One of great wealth [Old German]
Odin	Norse god of wisdom and death; inspiration, rage, frenzy [Old Norse/Old German]
Oengus	Irish form of Angus; one strength [Gaelic]
Ogden	From the surname; from the oak valley [Old English]
Olaf	Ancestor's relic [Old Norse]
Olav	Variant of Olaf; ancestor's relic [Old Norse]
Oleg	Holy [Russian]
Oli	Diminutive of Oliver; elf warrior [Old German]; Ancestor's descendant [Old Norse]
Olimpio	Of Mount Olympus [Greek]
Olin	He who inherits [Swedish/Norse]
Olo	Diminutive of Orlando, Italian form of Roland; famous across the land [Old German]
Oliver	Elf warrior [Old German]; Or ancestor's descendant [Old Norse]
Olivier	Elf warrior [Old German]; Or ancestor's descendant [Old Norse]
Ollie	Diminutive of Oliver; elf warrior [Old German]; Ancestor's descendant [Old Norse]
Olson	From the surname; Olaf's son; ancestor's relic [Old Norse]

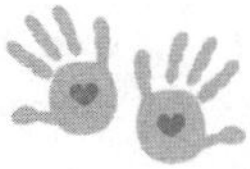

Olympos Of Mount Olympus [Greek]
Olympus Of Mount Olympus [Greek]
Omar Variant of Umar; flourishing, fruitful [Arabic]
Omri My sheaf; harvest [Hebrew]
Onslow From the surname; from the zealot's hill [Old English]
Ontario From the name of the region in Canada
Ora To pray; one who prays [atin]
Oral Eagle [Slavic]; speaker, word [Latin]
Oran Light [Aramaic]. Or little pale green one [Irish]
Orban Hungarian form of Urban; of the city [Latin]
Orfeo Italian form of Orpheus; darkness of night [Greek]
Orlando Italian form of Roland; famous across the land [Old German]
Ormond From the Irish surname; descendants of the red-haired [Gaelic]
Ormonde Variant of Ormond; descendants of the red-haired [Gaelic]
Orpheus Darkness of night [Greek]
Orrell From the surname; from the ore hill [Old English]
Orson From the surname; bear cub [Norman French]
Orton From the surname; variant of Horton; from the grey settlement [Old English]
Orval Variant of Orville; golden city [French]
Orville Golden city [French]. Invented by 18th century writer Fanny Eurney
Orwell From the surname; from a branch of the river [Old English]
Os Diminutive of names beginning with Os-
Osbert God bright [Old English]
Osborn God bear [Old English]
Osborne From the surname; variant of Osborn; god bear [Old English]
Osbourne From the surname; variant of Osborn; god bear [Old English]
Oscar Deer friend [Gaelic]; or god spear [Old English]
Osian Little deer [Welsh & Irish]
Osiris Of styrong eyesight [Egyptian]
Oskar Variant of Oscar; deer friend [Gaelic]. Or god spear [Old English]
Oslo From the name of the Norwegian city
Osmand Variant of Osmond; from the surname; with divine protection [Old English]
Osmond From the surname; with divine protection [Old English]
Oswald God's power [Old English]
Oswin God friend [Old English]
Otek Polish form of Otto; wealth; fortune [Old German]
Otis Variant of Otto; wealth; fortune [Old German]
Otto Wealth; fortune [Old German]
Owen Welsh form of Eugene; well-born [Greek]. Or youth [Welsh]
Oz Diminutive of names beginning with Os-
Ozzie Diminutive of names beginning with Os-
Ozzy Diminutive of names beginning with Os-

P

Pablo	Spanish form of Paul; humble one [Latin]
Pace	From the surname; peace [Old English]
Pacey	From the surname; from the French place name Pacy [Gaulish]
Paco	Eagle [Native American]
Padden	From the surname; a diminutive of Patrick; nobleman [Latin]
Paden	Diminutive of Padden/Patten/Patrick; nobleman [Latin]
Paddy	Diminutive of Patrick; nobleman [Latin]
Padraig	Irish form of Patrick; nobleman [Latin]
Pagan	Countryman; man from the country [Old English]
Page	From the surname; page; servant
Painter	From the surname; painter
Paisley	From the surname, or the name of the Scottish town; church; cemetry
Paladin	Of the palace; knightly title [French]
Palermo	From the name of the Sicilian city
Palin	From the surname; wine-bearer [Old English]
Palmer	From the surname; pilgrim [Latin]
Pancras	All power [Greek]
Parker	From the surname; park keeper
Parnell	From the surname; little Peter [Old French]
Parris	From the surname; from Paris, France
Parry	From the Welsh surname; son of Harry, diminutive of Henry; home ruler [German]
Parson	From the surname; clergyman [Old English]
Pascal	Easter [Old French]
Pasco	Cornish form of Pascal; easter [Old French]
Pat	Diminutive of Patrick; nobleman [Latin]
Paterson	From the surname; son of Peter; stone; rock [Greek]
Patrick	Nobleman [Latin]
Patsy	Diminutive of Patrick; nobleman [Latin]
Patton	From the surname; a diminutive of Patrick; nobleman [Latin]
Paul	Humble one [Latin]
Paulie	Diminutive of Paul; humble one [Latin]
Paxton	From the surname; from Pœcc's town [Old English]
Payton	Variant of Peyton; from the surname; from Paega's town [Old English]
Paz	Diminutive of Pazel; peace [Hebrew]
Pazel	Peace [Hebrew]
Peal	Variant of Peale; from the surname; bell ringer
Peale	From the surname; bell ringer

Pearce	Variant of Pierce; from the surname, derived from Piers/Peter; stone; rock [Greek]
Peers	Variant of Piers, medieval form of Peter; stone; rock [Greek]
Perce	Diminutive of Percy; from the surname; from Perci, Normandy
Percival	Form of Peredur; hard spears [Welsh]
Percy	From Perci, Normandy. Or diminutive of Percival; hard spears [Welsh]
Peredur	Hard spears [Welsh]
Peregrine	Traveller [Latin]
Perkin	Diminutive of Peter; little Peter; little rock [Greek]
Perkins	From the surname; little Peter; little rock [Greek]
Perran	Little dark one [Cornish]
Perry	Living near the pear tree [Old English]; or son of Herry/Henry [Welsh]
Perseus	To destroy [Greek]
Peru	From the name of the South American country
Petar	Variant of Peter; stone; rock [Greek]
Pete	Diminutive of Peter; stone; rock [Greek]
Peter	Stone; rock [Greek]
Peterson	From the surname; son of Peter; stone; rock [Greek]
Petey	Diminutive of Peter; stone; rock [Greek]
Peverell	From the surname; little boy; pepper [Latin]
Peyton	From the surname; from Paega's town [Old English]
Phil	Diminutive of Philip; friend of horses [Greek]
Philip	Friend of horses [Greek]
Phillip	Variant of Philip; friend of horses [Greek]
Philo	Loving [Greek]
Phineas	Oracle [Hebrew]
Phoenix	From the mythical bird reborn in fire [Greek]
Phyllon	Leaf [Greek]
Phylo	Variant of Philo; loving [Greek]
Picard	From the surname; from Picardy, France
Pierce	From the surname, derived from Piers/Peter; stone; rock [Greek]
Pierre	French form of Peter; stone; rock [Greek]
Piers	Medieval form of Peter; stone; rock [Greek]
Pieter	Variant of Peter; stone; rock [Greek]
Pike	From the name of the fish; or from the surname
Pilot	Pilot
Pine	From the name of the tree
Pip	Diminutive of Philip; friend of horses [Greek]
Placido	Quiet; calm [Latin]
Porter	From the surname; door keeper [Latin]
Porthos	From a character in Dumas's The Three Musketeers
Portland	From the surname or place name; land near the port
Potter	From the surname; one who makes or sells pots/pottery
Powell	From the surname; son of Howell
Power	Power

Powers From the surname; power
Prentice From the surname; apprentice
Prentis Variant of Prentice; from the surname; apprentice
Prescott From the surname; from the priest's cottage [Old English]
Presley From the surname; from the priest clearing [Old English]
Preston From the surname; from Preston; priest town [Old English]
Prewitt From the surname; brave little one [Old French]
Prince Prince; royal title [Latin]
Prosper Fortunate, successful [Latin]
Pry Diminutive of Pryor; from the surname; prior
Pryor From the surname; prior
Ptolemy Warlike [Greek]
Purcell From the surname, a variant of Percival; hard spears [Old German]
Purdie From the surname; by God [Norman French]

Q

Quade From the surname; born fourth
Quaid Variant of Quade; from the surname; born fourth
Quartz From the name of the mineral
Quebec From the name of the Canadian city
Quennel From the surname; from the little oak tree [Old French]
Quentin Fifth; fifth child; child born in fifth month, or on fifth of the month
Quest Quest; mission; purpose
Quigley From the surname; from the maternal side [Irish/Old Norse]
Quillan From the surname; cub [Irish]
Quimby From the surname; from the woman's estate [Old Norse]
Quin Variant of Quinn; from the surname; chief [Irish]
Quincey Variant of Quincy; from the surname derived from Quintus; fifth [Latin]
Quincy From the surname derived from Quintus; fifth [Latin]
Quinlan From the Irish surname; slender [Gaelic]
Quinn From the surname; chief [Irish]
Quint Diminutive of Quentin/Quinton
Quinten Variant of Quentin; fifth; fifth child; child born in fifth month, or on fifth of the month
Quintin Variant of Quentin; fifth; fifth child; child born in fifth month, or on fifth of the month
Quinton Variant of Quentin; fifth; fifth child; child born in fifth month, or on fifth of the month
Quixote From the surname; thigh; thigh armour; hip [Spanish]

R

Rab	Scots diminutive of Robert; bright fame [Old German]
Rabbie	Scots diminutive of Robert; bright fame [Old German]
Rad	Advisor
Radcliff	From the surname; from the red cliff [Old English]
Radclyffe	From the surname; variant of Rsdciff; from the red cliff [Old English]
Radley	From the surname; from the red meadow
Raeburn	From the surname; from the stream where does drink [Old English]
Rafe	Variant of Ralph, reflecting pronouciation; counsel of the wolf [Old Norse]
Rafferty	From the Irish surname; flood tide [Irish]
Rafael	Variant of Raphael; God has healed [Hebrew]
Ragnar	Warrior of judgement [Old Norse]
Raimond	Variant of Raymond; wise protector [Old German]
Rain	Rain
Rainar	Wise army [Old German]
Rainier	Wise army [Old German]
Rajiv	Striped [Sanskrit]
Raleigh	From the red clearing; or from the roe deer clearing [Old English]
Ralf	Variant of Ralph; counsel of the wolf [Old Norse]
Ralph	Counsel of the wolf [Old Norse]
Ralphie	Diminutive of Ralph; counsel of the wolf [Old Norse]
Ramsay	Variant of Ramsey; from the surname; from the wild-garlic island [Old English]
Ramsey	From the surname; from the wild-garlic island [Old English]
Randal	Variant of Randall; shield rim of the wolf [Old German]
Randall	From the surname derived from Randel; shield rim of the wolf [Old German]
Randell	Medieval diminutive of Randolph; shield rim of the wolf [Old German]
Randell	Variant of Randall; shield rim of the wolf [Old German]
Randolf	Shield rim of the wolf [Old German]
Randolph	Variant of Randolph; shield rim of the wolf [Old German]
Randy	Diminutive of Randall or Randolf; shiled rim of the wolf [Old German]
Raoul	French form of Ralph; counsel of the wolf [Old Norse]
Raphael	God has healed [Hebrew]
Rastus	Short form of Erastus; beloved [Greek]
Raven	From the name of the bird [Old English]
Ray	Diminutive of Raymond; wise protector [Old German]. Or ray; beam of light
Rayburn	Variant of Raeburn; from the stream where does drink [Old English]
Raymond	Wise protector [Old German]
Raymund	Variant of Raymond; wise protector [Old German]

Raynard	Variant of Reynard; brave counsellor [Old German]
Rayner	War counsellor [Old German
Read	Variant of Reed; red-haired one; person living in a wood clearing [Old English]
Reagan	From the Irish surname; impulsive [Irish]
Reason	Reason
Reave	Variant of Reeve; from the surname; bailiff [Old English]
Reb	Diminutive of Rebel; rebel
Rebel	Rebel
Red	From the colour; person with red hair pr ruddy complexion
Redd	Variant of Red; from the colour; person with red hair pr ruddy complexion
Redford	From the surnmae; from the red ford [Old English]
Reece	Variant of Rhys; ardour; enthusiasm [Welsh]
Reed	From the surname; red-haired one; person living in a wood clearing [Old English]
Reese	Variant of Rhys; ardour; enthusiasm [Welsh]
Reeve	From the surname; bailiff [Old English]
Reg	Diminutive of Reginald; wise ruler [Old German]
Reggie	Diminutive of Reginald; wise ruler [Old German]
Reginald	Variant of Reynold; wise ruler [Old German]
Reid	Variant of Reed; red-haired one; person living in a wood clearing [Old English]
Reilly	From a small stream; or courageous [Gaelic]; from a rye clearing [Old English]
Rembrandt	Wise swordsman [Old German]
Remington	From the surname; from the settlement on the river bank [Old English]
Renaud	French form of Reginald; wise ruler [Old German]
Rene	English form of René; born again [Latin]
René	Born again [Latin]
Reuben	Behold, a son [Hebrew]
Rex	King [Latin]
Reynard	Brave cousellor [Old German]
Reynold	Wise ruler [Old German]
Rhett	From a Dutch surname; adviser
Rhodri	Wheel; circle [Welsh]
Rhys	Ardour; enthusiasm [Welsh]
Rian	Variant of Ryan; little king [Gaelic]
Ricardo	Latin form of Richard; brave, powerful one [Old German]
Rich	Diminutive of Richard; brave, powerful one [Old German]
Richard	Brave, powerful one [Old German]
Richie	Diminutive of Richard; brave, powerful one [Old German]
Richmond	powerful protector [Old German]. Or from the surname/place name
Rick	Diminutive of Richard; brave, powerful one [Old German]
Rickey	Diminutive of Richard; brave, powerful one [Old German]
Ricki	Diminutive of Richard; brave, powerful one [Old German]
Rickie	Diminutive of Richard; brave, powerful one [Old German]
Ricky	Diminutive of Richard; brave, powerful one [Old German]
Ridley	From the surname; from the reed clearing; from the cleared wood [Old English]

Rigby From the surname; from the ridge farm [Old Norse]
Riley From a small stream; or courageous [Gaelic]; from a rye clearing [Old English]
Ringo Nickname
Riordan Bard; royal poet [Irish]
Ripley From the surname; from the strip clearing [Old English]
Ritchie Variant of Richie; diminutive of Richard; brave, powerful one [Old German]
River River
Rob Diminutive of Robert; bright fame [Old German]
Robbie Diminutive of Robert; bright fame [Old German]
Robby Diminutive of Robert; bright fame [Old German]
Robert Bright fame [Old German]
Robin Diminutive of Robert; bright fame [Old German]
Rocco Rest [Italian/German]
Rochester From the surname; from the stone camp or fortress [Old English]
Rocky Diminutive of Rocco; rest [Old German]
Rod Famous power [Old German]. Or of Rodney; from Hroda's island [Old English]
Roddy Famous power [Old German]. Or of Rodney; from Hroda's island [Old English]
Roderick Famous power [Old German]
Rodge Diminutive of Rodger/Roger; famous spear [Old German]
Rodger Variant of Roger; famous spear [Old German]
Rodney From the surname; from Hroda's island [Old English]
Rodolph Variant of Rudolf; famous wolf [Old German]
Roger Famous spear [Old German]
Roland Famous across the land; famously brave [Old German]
Rolf A contgracted form of Rudolf; famous wolf [Old German]
Rolland Variant of Roland; famous across the land; famously brave [Old German]
Rollo Latinized form of Rolf. contgracted form of Rudolf; famous wolf [Old German]
Rolo Variant of Rollo; Latinized form of Rolf. Famous wolf [Old German]
Rolph Contracted form of Rudolf; famous wolf [Old German]
Roly Diminutive of Roland; famous across the land; famously brave [Old German]
Ron Diminutive of Ronald; wise ruler [Old Norse]
Ronald Wise ruler [Old Norse]
Ronan Little seal [Irish]
Ronnie Diminutive of Ronald; wise ruler [Old Norse]
Ronny Diminutive of Ronald; wise ruler [Old Norse]
Roosevelt From the surname; rose field [Dutch]
Rory English form of Ruaidhri; red king [Gaelic]
Roscoe From the surname; from the doe wood [Old Norse]
Ross From Ross, northern Scotland; from the promontory or headland [Gaelic]
Roswell From the horse spring [Old English]
Rowan From the name of the tree. Or from the surname; red-haired one [Gaelic]
Rowland Variant of Roland; famous across the land; famously brave [Old German]
Rowley Diminutive of Roland; famous across the land; famously brave [Old German]
Roy Red-haired; ruddy-complexioned [Gaelic]. Or king [Norman French]

Royal	Royal; of royal blood
Royale	Variant of Royal; royal; of royal blood
Royce	From the surname; derived from a variant of Rose; from the name of the flower
Roydon	From the surname; from the rye hill [Old English]
Royle	From the surname; from the rye hill [Old English]
Royston	From the surname; from the town of Royse; Rose's town [Old English]
Ruaidhri	Red king [Gaelic]
Rube	Diminutive of Reuben; behold, a son [Hebrew]
Rudolph	English form of Rudolf; famous wolf [Old German]
Rudy	Diminutive of Rudolf; famous wolf [Old German]
Rudyard	From a red yard [Old English]
Rufus	Red-haired [Latin]
Rupert	German variant form of Robert; bright fame [Old German]
Russ	Diminutive of Russell; from the surname; little red one [French]
Russel	Variant of Russell; from the surname; little red one [French]
Russell	From the surname; little red one [French]
Rusty	From a nickname; reddish or rusty haired one
Ryan	From the surname; little king [Gaelic]
Ryder	From thel surname; mounted warrior; messenger [Old English]
Ryker	Variant of the German surname Riker; rich [Old German]
Rylan	Variant of the English surname Ryland; from the rye land [Old English]
Ryley	From a small stream; or courageous [Gaelic]; from a rye clearing [Old English]

S

Saban	Variant of Sabin; of the Sabines [Latin]
Sabastian	Variant of Sebastian; from Sebaste, Asia Minor [Latin]
Sabin	Of the Sabines [Latin]
Sacheverell	From the surname; derived from a Norman place name
Sachie	Diminutive of Sacheverell
Sagan	Variant of Sage; From the herb. Or wise person
Sage	From the herb. Or wise person
Sal	Diminutive of Salvador and other names beginning with Sal-
Salman	Safety [Arabic]
Salo	Diminutive of Solomon/Saloman; peace [Hebrew]
Saloman	Variant of Solomon; peace [Hebrew]
Salvador	Saviour [Spanish/Latin]
Salvator	Saviour [Latin]
Sam	Diminutive of Samuel; name of God; God has heardd. Or of Samson; sun [Hebrew]

Sammie	Diminutive of of Samuel; name of God [Hebrew]. Or of Samson; sun [Hebrew]
Sammy	Diminutive of of Samuel; name of God [Hebrew]. Or of Samson; sun [Hebrew]
Sampson	Variant of Samson; sun [Hebrew]
Samson	Sun [Hebrew]
Samuel	Name of God; God has heard [Hebrew]
Sandford	From the surname; variant of Sanford; from a sandy ford [Old English]
Sandy	Diminutive of Alexander; the defender [Greek]. Or sandy-coloured
Sanford	From the surname; from a sandy ford [Old English]
Santana	Contraction of Santa Ana [Spanish]
Santiago	From the Chilean city, or saint's name; St. James; supplanter [Hebrew]
Santos	Saint; holy [Spanish/Latin]
Sarkis	Protector; shepherd [Armenian]
Sasha	Russian and Ukrainian diminutive of Alexander; the defender [Greek]
Satchel	From the surname; bag maker [Old English]
Sawyer	From the surname; one who saws wood [Old English]
Saxon	From the surname; of the Saxons; knife [Old German]
Sayer	From the surname; reciter; woodcutter [Old English]
Sayre	Variant of Sayer; from the surname; reciter; woodcutter [Old English]
Schuyler	From the surname; scholar [Dutch]
Scot	Variant of Scott; from the surname; Scottish person; Gaelic speaker
Scott	From the surname; Scottish person; Gaelic speaker
Scottie	Diminutive of Scott; from the surname; Scottish person; Gaelic speaker
Scotty	Diminutive of Scott; from the surname; Scottish person; Gaelic speaker
Seamus	Irish form of James; supplanter [Hebrew]
Sean	Irish form of John; God is gracious [Hebrew]
Seb	Diminutive of Sebastian; from Sebaste, Asia Minor [Latin]
Sebastian	From Sebaste, Asia Minor [Latin]
Sebastien	Variant of Sebastian; from Sebaste, Asia Minor [Latin]
Sedric	Variant of Cedric; love [Celtic]
Seeger	From the surnmae; seaman [Old English]
Sefton	From the surname; from the settlement in the rushes [Old English]
Selby	From the surname; from Selby; from the willow farm [Old Norse]
Selwyn	Friend of the house/castle/manor [Old English]
Semon	Greek variant of Simon; he has heard [Hebrew]
Semyon	Russian form of Simon; he has heard [Hebrew]
September	From the name of the month
Sequoia	From the name of the Californian tree [Cherokee]
Sergei	Russian form of the Roman family name Sergius; servant [Latin]
Serges	French form of the Roman family name Sergius; servant [Latin]
Seth	Appointed [Hebrew]
Seward	From the surname; guardian of victory [Old English]
Seymour	From the surname; from the French town of Saint Maur
Shad	Perhaps a variant of Chad; battle [Welsh]
Shain	Variant of Shane/Sean, Irish form of John; God is gracious [Hebrew]

Shamus	Anglicized form of Seamus, Irish form of James; supplanter [Hebrew]
Shane	Anglicized form of Sean, Irish form of John; God is gracious [Hebrew]
Shannon	From the name of the River Shannon
Shanon	Variant of Shannon; from the name of the River Shannon
Shaquille	Variant of Shakil; handsome [Arabic]
Shaun	Anglicized form of Sean, Irish form of John; God is gracious [Hebrew]
Shaw	From the surname; from the thicket [Old English]
Shawn	Anglicized form of Sean, Irish form of John; God is gracious [Hebrew]
Shayne	Variant of Shane/Sean, Irish form of John; God is gracious [Hebrew]
Sheard	Gap between hills [Old English]
Shel	Diminutive of Sheldon; from the surname; from the steep valley [Old English]
Shelby	Variant of Selby; from the surname; from Selby; from the willow farm [Old Norse]
Sheldon	From the surname; from the steep valley [Old English]
Shelley	From the surname; from the clearing on the bank [Old English]
Shelly	Variant of Shelley; from the surname; from the clearing on the bank [Old English]
Shelton	From the surname; from the shelf town [Old English]
Sheridan	From the Irish surname;searcher [Gaelic]
Sherlock	Fair-haired [Old English]
Sherman	From the surname; shear man; one who cuts cloth [Old English]
Sherwood	From the surname; from Sherwood; from the bright forest
Shirley	From the surname; from the bright clearing [Old English]
Sid	Diminutive of Sidney; from the surname; from a wide island [Old English]
Sidney	From the surname; from a wide island [Old English]
Sigmund	Victory protector [Old German/Old Norse]
Silas	From the forest [Latin]. Or Greek form of Saul; prayed for [Hebrew]
Silver	Silver; from the precious metal or colour
Silvester	Of the forest [Latin]
Simon	He has heard [Hebrew]
Sinclair	From the surname; from the Norman French town Saint Clair
Sinjin	Variant of the name St. John; God is gracious [Hebrew]
Skylar	Variant of Skyler/Schulyer; scholar [Dutch]
Skyler	Variant of Schulyer; scholar [Dutch]
Slade	From the surname; from the valley [Old English]
Sly	Diminutive of Silvester; of the forest [Latin]
Smith	From the surname; metal worker, blacksmith [Old English]
Sol	Diminutive of Solomon; peace [Hebrew]
Solomon	Peace [Hebrew]
Sonnie	Variant of Sonny; from a nickname; son; lad; young boy
Sonny	From a nickname; son; lad; young boy
Sparrow	From the name of the bird [Old English]
Spencer	From the surname; dispenser, i.e. of provisions [English]
Spike	From a nickname; one with spiky hair
Stacey	Variant of Stacy; from the surname; fruitful [Greek]
Stacy	From the surname; fruitful [Greek]

Stafford	From the surname; from Stafford; from the landing ford [Old English]
Stan	Diminutive of Stanley; from the surname; stone clearing [Old English]
Stanford	From the surname; from Stanford; from the stone ford [Old English]
Stanley	From the surname; stone clearing [Old English]
Ste	Diminutive of Stephen; crown; honour; reward [Greek]
Steph	Diminutive of Stephen; crown; honour; reward [Greek]
Stephen	Crown; honour; reward [Greek]
Sterling	From the Scottish surname; from Stirling. Or sterling, excellent
Steve	Diminutive of Stephen; crown; honour; reward [Greek]
Steven	Variant of Stephen; crown; honour; reward [Greek]
Stevie	Diminutive of Stephen; crown; honour; reward [Greek]
Stew	Diminutive of Stewart; steward; house guard [Old English]
Stewart	Steward; house guard [Old English]
Stirling	From the Scottish surname; variant of Sterling; from Stirling
Storm	Storm; tempest
Stu	Short form of Stuart/Stewart; steward; house guard [Old English]
Stuart	Variant of Stewart; steward; house guard [Old English]
Sullivan	From the Irish surname; little dark eye [Irish]
Syd	Short form of Sydney; from a wide island [Old English]. Or for the Australian city
Sydney	Variant of Sydney; from a wide island [Old English]. Or for the Australian city
Sylvester	Variant of Silvester; of the forest [Latin]

T

Tad	Diminutive of Thaddeus, a form of Theodore; gift of God [Greek]
Taegan	Variant of Teagan; from the Irish surname; little poet [Gaelic]
Talbot	From the surname; message of destruction [Old German]
Talon	Talon, claw, ankle bone [Latin]
Tanner	From the surname; one who tans hides
Tate	From the surname, deriving from old English name Tata; unknown meaning
Tatton	From the surname; from Tata's town [Old English]
Tayler	Variant of Taylor; from the surname; tailor [Latin]
Taylor	From the surname; tailor
Teagan	From the Irish surname; little poet [Gaelic]
Ted	Diminutive of Edward; wealthy guard. Or of Theodore; gift of God [Greek]
Teddy	Diminutive of Edward; wealthy guard. Or of Theodore; gift of God [Greek]
Tel	Diminutive of Terence. Or of Terry, a form of Thiery; ruler of the people [Greek]
Temple	From the surname; one associated with the Knights Templar

Tennyson	From an English surname; son of Tenney/ Dennis; god from Nysa [Greek]
Terance	Variant of Terence; from the Roman family name Terentius
Terell	Variant of Terrell; nickname for a stubborn person [Norman French]
Terence	From the Roman family name Terentius
Terrance	Variant of TERENCE.
Terrell	From the surname; from a nickname for a stubborn person [Norman French]
Terrence	Variant of Terence; from the Roman family name Terentius
Terry	Form of Thiery/ Theodoric; ruler of the people [Greek]; or diminutive of Terence
Tex	From a nickname; person from Texas, USA
Thad	Diminutive of Thaddeus, a form of Theodore; gift of God [Greek]
Thaddeus	Form of Theodore; gift of God [Greek]
Thane	From the old noble title thegn [Old English]
Theo	Diminutive of Theodore; gift of God [Greek]. Or of Theobald; bold people [German]
Theobald	Bold people [Old German]
Theodore	Gift of God [Greek]
Thiago	Variant of Tiago, a diminutive of Santiago/Saint James; supplanter [Hebrew]
Thom	Diminutive of Thomas; twin [Aramaic/Greek]
Thomas	Twin [Aramaic/Greek]
Thorburn	From the surname; Thor's bear [Old Norse]
Thorley	From the surname; from the thorn clearing [Old English]
Thornton	From the surname; from Thornton; from the thorn town [Old English]
Thurstan	From the surname; Thor's stone [Old Norse]
Tiago	Diminutive of Santiago/Saint James; supplanter [Hebrew]
Tibby	Diminutive of Theobald; bold peole [Old German]
Tierney	From the surname; lord [Irish]
Tiger	Tiger
Tim	Diminutive of Timothy; honouring God [Greek]
Timmy	Diminutive of Timothy; honouring God [Greek]
Timothy	Honouring God [Greek]
Titus	Title of honour; defender [Latin]
Tobias	God is good [Hebrew]
Tobin	From an English surname derived from Tobias; God is good [Hebrew]
Toby	Medieval form of Tobias; God is good [Hebrew]
Tod	Variant of Todd; fox [Old English]
Todd	Fox [Old English]
Tolly	Diminutive of Bartholomew; son of Talmai; furrowed [Hebrew]
Tom	Diminutive of Thomas; twin [Aramaic/Greek]
Tommie	Diminutive of Thomas; twin [Aramaic/Greek]
Tommy	Diminutive of Thomas; twin [Aramaic/Greek]
Tony	Diminutive of Anthony; priceless; handsome [Etruscan]
Topher	Diminutive of Christopher; bearing Christ; carrying Christ [Greek]
Trace	Diminutive of Tracy; from a Norman place name; domain of Thracius [French]
Tracey	Variant of Tracy; from a Norman place name; domain of Thracius [French]
Tracy	From the surname; from a Norman place name; domain of Thracius [French]

Trafford	From the surname; from Trafford; from the fishtrap ford [Old English]
Tranter	From the surname; wagoner [Old English]
Travers	From the surname; from the crossing place, bridge or ford [Old French/Latin]
Travis	Variant of Travers; from the crossing place, bridge or ford [Old French/Latin]
Trent	From the surname; one who lives by the River Trent in England
Trenton	From the name of the New Jersey city;Trent's town
Trev	Diminutive of Trevor; from the surname; from the large village [Welsh]
Trevelyan	From the surname; from thehome on the hill [Cornish]
Trevor	From the surname; from the large village [Welsh]
Trey	From a nickname meaning three
Tristan	French form of Drustan; tumultuous [Pictish]
Tristen	Variant of Tristan/Drustan; tumultuous [Pictish]
Tristin	Variant of Tristan/Drustan; tumultuous [Pictish]
Triston	Variant of Tristan/Drustan; tumultuous [Pictish]
Tristram	Variant of Tristan/Drustan; tumultuous [Pictish]
Troy	From the surname; from Troyes, France. Or for the ancient city of Troy
Trueman	From the surname; variant of Truman; trusty man [Old English]
Truman	From the surname; trusty man [Old English]
Tucker	From the surname; one who tucks/fulls cloth [Old English]
Ty	Diminutive of names beginning with Ty
Tye	From the surname; pasture [Old English]
Tylar	Variant of Tyler; from the surname; roof tiler
Tyler	From the surname; roof tiler
Tylor	Variant of Tyler; from the surname; roof tiler
Tyrell	Variant of Terrell; nickname for a stubborn person [Norman French]
Tyron	Variant of Tyrone; from the name of the Northern Irish county
Tyrone	From the name of the Northern Irish county
Tyrrell	Variant of Terrell; nickname for a stubborn person [Norman French]
Tyson	Nickname for a quarrelsome person; firebrand [Norman French]

U

Ubert	Spanish form of Hubert; bright heart [Old German]
Ulric	Wealthy, powerful ruler [Old German]
Ulysses	Latin form of Odysseus; to hate [Greek]
Umberto	Famous warrior [Old German]
Upton	From the surname; from the upper town [Old English]
Upwood	From the surname; from the upper wood
Urbain	French form of Urban; of the city [Latin]

Urban Of the city [Latin]
Urbano Portuguese form of Urban; of the city [Latin]
Urbanus Variant of Urban; of the city [Latin]
Uri My light [Hebrew]
Uriah God is my light [Hebrew]
Usain Beautiful [Arabic]
Usher From the surname; usher; doorkeeper [Norman French]

V

Vadim Attractive [Russian]
Val Diminutive of Valentine; strong; vigorous [Latin]
Valdemar Scandinavian variant of Vladimir; famous prince [Slavic]
Valentine Strong; vigorous [Latin]
Van Diminutive of names containing -van-
Vance From the surname; from the marsh [Old English]
Vaughn From the Welsh surname; little [Welsh]
Vere From the surname; from the place of alder trees [Norman French/Gaulish]
Vergil Variant of Virgil; from the Roman family name Vergilius
Vern Short form of Vernon;
Vernon From the surname; from the place of alder trees [Norman French/Gaulish]
Vic Diminutive of Victor; victor [Latin]
Victor Victor [Latin]
Vikram Brave [Hindi]
Viktor Variant of Victor; victor [Latin]
Villem Variant of William; resolute protector [Old German]
Villiers From the surname; town dwellers [French]
Vin Diminutive of Vincent; to conquer [Latin]
Vinal From the surname; from the vine hall [Old English]
Vince Diminutive of Vincent; to conquer [Latin]
Vincent To conquer [Latin]
Vinnie Diminutive of Vincent; to conquer [Latin]
Vinny Diminutive of Vincent; to conquer [Latin]
Virgil From the Roman family name Vergilius
Vitale Variant of Vito; alive [Latin]
Vito Alive [Latin]
Vivian Alive [Latin]
Vladimir Famous prince [Slavic]
Vladislav Glorious ruler [Slavic]

W

Wade	From the surname; from the ford; or to go [Old English]
Waldo	To rule [Old German]
Walker	From the surname; one who fulls/tucks/walks cloth [Old English]
Wallace	From the surname; foreigner; Welsh [Norman French]
Wallis	From the surname, a variant of Wallace; foreigner; Welsh [Norman French]
Wally	Ruler of the army [Old German]. Or of Wallace; foreigner; Welsh [Norman French]
Walt	Diminutive of Walter; ruler of the army [Old German]
Walter	Ruler of the army [Old German]
Walton	From the surname; from the stream town, wood town, or wall town [Old English]
Ward	From the surname; guard; watchman [Old English]
Wardell	From the surname; from the watch hill [Old English]
Warner	From the surname, derived from Werner; army guard [Old German]
Warren	Animal enclosure [Norman French]; from the town of La Varenne, Normandy.
Warrick	Variant of Warwick; from Warwick; from the dam settlement [Old English]
Warwick	From the surname; from Warwick; from the dam settlement [Old English]
Washington	From the surname; from Washington, England
Wat	Diminutive of Walter; ruler of the army [Old German]
Wayland	Form of Weland; land skilled [Old English]
Waylon	Variant of Wayland/Weland; land skilled [Old English]
Wayne	From the surname; wagon maker [Old English]
Webster	From the surname; weaver [Old English]
Weldon	From the surname; from the hill near a spring [Old English]
Wendell	From the surname derived from Wendel; of the Vandals
Wes	Diminutive of Wesley; from the surname; from the west meadow [Old English]
Wesley	From the surname; from the west meadow [Old English]
Westley	Variant of Wesley; from the surname; from the west meadow [Old English]
Weston	From the surname; from the west town [Old English]
Whitaker	From the surname; from thewhite field [Old English]
Whitney	From the surname; from the white island [Old English]
Wil	Diminutive of William and other names beginning with Wil-
Wilbur	From the surname; wild boar [Old English]
Wilburn	From the surname; uncertain meaning
Wiley	From the surname; from the temple clearing [Old English]. Or wily; cunning
Wilf	Diminutive of Wilfred; desiting peace [Old English]
Wilford	From the surname; from the willow ford [Old English]
Wilfred	Desiring peace [Old English]
Wilfrid	Variant of Wilfred; desiting peace [Old English]

Wilkie Derived from a diminutive of William; resolute protector [Old German]

Will Diminutive of William; resolute protector [Old German].

Willard From the English surname, derived from Willihard; brave desire [Old German]

William Resolute protector [Old German]

Willie Diminutive of William; resolute protector [Old German]

Willis Derived from Will, diminutive of William; resolute protector [Old German]

Willoughby From the surname; from the willow town [Old English]

Willy Diminutive of William; resolute protector [Old German]

Wilmer From the surname; will to be famous [Old German]

Wilson From the surname; son of William; resolute protector [Old German]

Wilt Diminutive of Wilton; from willow town, well town or the town on the River Wylye

Wilton From Wilton; from willow town, well town or the town on the River Wylye

Windsor From the surname; from Windsor; riverbank with a windlass [Old English]

Winfred Friend of peace [Old English]

Winslow From the surname; from Wine's hill [Old English]

Winston From the surname; from Winston, England

Winthrop From the surname; from Winthrop, England [Old English]

Winton From the surname; from Wine's enclosure [Old English]

Wisdom Wisdom

Wolf Wolf; or diminutive of Germanic names e.g. Wolfgang, Wolfram etc.

Wolfe Variant of Wolf; wolf; or diminutive of Germanic names e.g. Wolfgang, Wolfram etc.

Woodrow From the surname; from the row of houses by a wood [Old English]

Woody Diminutive of Woodrow; or nickname from wood

Wright From the surname; craftsman [Old English]

Wyatt From the surname; battle brave [Old English]

Wynne From the surname derived from the old given name Wine; friend [Old English]

Wystan Battle stone [Old English]

X

Xander Diminutive of Alexander; the defender [Greek]

Xavier New house [Basque]

Xavior Variant of Xavier; new house [Basque]

Xzavier Variant of Xavier; new house [Basque]

Y

Yakov	Supplanter [Hebrew]
Yancy	From the surname, taken fromf the Dutch name Jansen; Jans son
Yorick	Altered form of Scandinavian Jorg; George; farmer
York	From the surname; from York
Yuri	Russian form of George; farmer [Greek]

Z

Zac	Diminutive of Zachary; English form of Zacharias; God remembers [Hebrew]
Zach	Diminutive of Zachary; English form of Zacharias; God remembers [Hebrew]
Zachariah	God remembers [Hebrew]
Zachary	English form of Zacharias; God remembers [Hebrew]
Zachery	Variant of of Zachary; God remembers [Hebrew]
Zack	Diminutive of Zachary; English form of Zacharias; God remembers [Hebrew]
Zackary	Variant of of Zachary; God remembers [Hebrew]
Zackery	Variant of of Zachary; God remembers [Hebrew]
Zain	Variant of Zayn; beauty; grace [Arabic]
Zak	Diminutive of Zachary; English form of Zacharias; God remembers [Hebrew]
Zander	Diminutive of Alexander; the defender [Greek]
Zane	Possible variant of John; God is gracious [Hebrew]
Zavier	Variant of Xavier; new house [Basque]
Zayn	Beauty; grace [Arabic]
Zechariah	God remembers [Hebrew]
Zed	Diminutive of Zedekiah; justice of God {Hebrew]
Zedekiah	Justice of God {Hebrew]
Zeke	Diminutive of Ezekiel; God strenghens [Hebrew]
Zeph	Diminutive of Zephaniah; God has hidden [Hebrew]

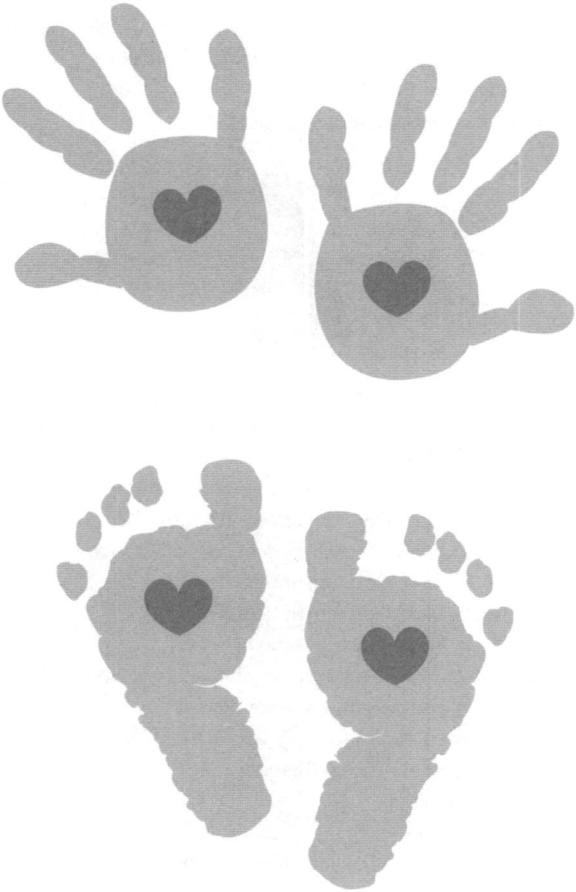

100 Popular *Girls* Names

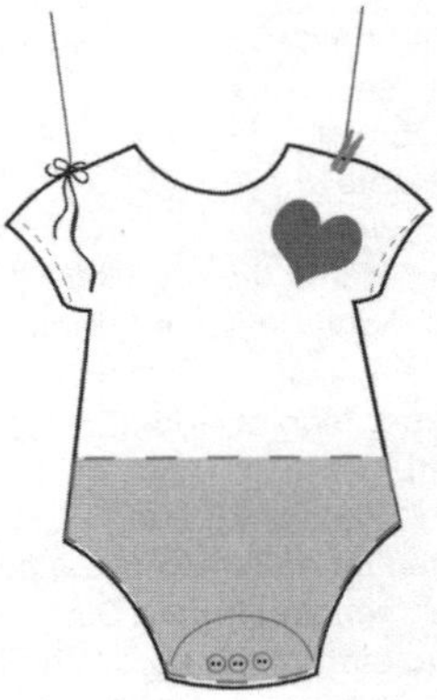

100 Popular Girls Names

Olivia	Variant of Olive; olive. Or feminine form of Oliver; elf warrior [Old German]
Ava	Variant of Eve; to breathe
Emma	Whole; universal [Old German]
Isabella	Latin form of Isabel; western form of Elizabeth; oath of God [Hebrew]
Sophia	Woman of wisdom [Greek]
Emily	Rival [Latin]
Mia	Diminutive of Maria; sea of sorrow; wished-for child [Greek]. Mine [Italian]
Charlotte	Feminine diminutive of Charles; warrior [Old German]
Amelia	Industrious, striving [Old German]
Aria	Song [Italian]
Harper	From the surname; one who plays or makes harps
Ella	Other [Norman French]. Or diminutive of Eleanor, Ellen etc.
Abigail	Father's joy [Hebrew]
Evelyn	From the surname; desired [Old German]
Lily	From the flower, symbolizing purity
Madison	From the surname; son of Maud
Avery	From the surname; powerful [old German]
Scarlett	From the surname; person who makes/sells scarlet clothes
Mila	Gracious; dear [Slavic]
Layla	Night [Arabic]
Grace	The virtue, grace [Latin]
Riley	From a small stream; or courageous [Gaelic]; from a rye clearing [English]
Chloe	Green shoot [Greek]
Ellie	Diminutive of Eleanor, Ellen etc.
Zoe	Life [Greek]
Aubrey	Feminine variant of Alberich; powerful [old German]
Penelope	Duck; weaver [Greek]
Elizabeth	Oath of God [Hebrew]
Hannah	Grace; favour [Hebrew]
Jessica	To behold [Hebrew]
Victoria	Feminine form of Victor; victory, victor [Latin]
Nora	Form of Eleanor; light; radiance [Arabic]. Or of Honora; the virtue of honour
Stella	Star [Latin]
Addison	From the surname; "son of Adam"
Luna	The moon [Latin]
Lucy	English form of Lucia; light [Latin]
Esmée	Feminine only variant of Esmé; loved; esteemed [old French]
Skylar	Variant of Skyler; scholar; from a Dutch surname
Natalie	Variant ofNatalia; birth of the Lord; Christmas Day [Latin]
Paisley	From the surname; from the Scottish town Paisley
Savannah	Grassy plain. Or from Savannah, Georgia, USA
Camilla	Unblemished virgin; ceremonial attendant [Latin]
Lillian	Form of Lily; the flower. Or diminutive of Elizabeth; oath of God [Hebrew]
Maya	Variant of Maia; the Roman goddess. From the Mayan people of America
Bella	Beautiful [Italian]; or diminutive of Isabella etc.
Brooklyn	Area of New York City
Audrey	Noble; strength [old English]
Leah	Weary [Hebrew]
Aaliyah	Feminine form of Aali/Ali; lofty, sublime [Arabic]
Hazel	Hazel tree, or the nut colour

Aurora	Dawn [Latin]
Poppy	From the name of the flower
Eva	Latin form of Eve; breathe; live [Hebrew]
Elena	Variant of Helen; torch [Greek]
Claire	Variant of Clara; clear; famous [Latin]
Eleanor	Light, radiance [Arabic]. Or variant of Helen; torch [Greek]
Adeline	Noble, diminutive of Adele
Madelyn	Variant of Madeline/Magdalen; from the village of Magdala on the Sea of Galilee
Kennedy	From the surname; armoured head [Gaelic]
Violet	From the name of the flower
Anna	Favour; grace [Hebrew]
Emilia	Variant of Emily; rival [Latin]
Maria	Sea of sorrow; bitter; wished-for child [Greek]
Hailey	Variant of Hayley; from the surname; of the hay clearing [Old English]
Kinsley	From the surname; royal victory [Old English]
Alice	Noble one; variant of Adelaide [Greek]
Gabriella	God is my strength [Hebrew]
Sadie	Diminutive of Sarah; lady; princess [Hebrew]
Arianna	Latin form of Ariadne; most holy [Greek]
Sarah	Lady; princess [Hebrew]
Isabelle	French form of Isabel; western form of Elizabeth; oath of God [Hebrew]
Peyton	From the English surname; from Paega's town [Old English]
Sophie	French form of Sophia; woman of wisdom [Greek]
Isla	Variant of Islay; from the Scottish island
Nevaeh	Heaven, spelled backwards
Clara	Clear; famous [Latin]
Serenity	Tranquility [Latin]
Kaylee	Kay + -lee
Eliana	My God has answered [Hebrew]. From the Roman family name Aelius; sun [Greek]
Alexa	A derivative of Alexandra; the defender [Greek]
Mackenzie	From the surname; son of the handsome one [Gaelic]
Everly	From the surname; from the boar meadow [Old English]
Reagan	From the Irish surname; impulsive [Irish]
Piper	One who plays the pipe or flute
Gianna	Diminutive of Giovanna or Joanna; God is gracious [Hebrew]
Daisy	From the flower
Julia	Feminine form of Julius; downy-bearded [Greek]
Willow	From the name of the tree
Autumn	Autumn
Caroline	Warrior [Old German]
Samantha	Feminine form of Samuel; God has heard [Hebrew}] + -antha; flower [Greek]
Quinn	From the Irish surname; descendant of the chief [Irish]
Naomi	Pleasantness [Hebrew]
Ruby	From the name of the precious stone; red
Cora	Maiden [Greek]
Melanie	Dark; black [Latin]
Delilah	Delicate; languishing [Hebrew]
Phoebe	Bright, pure one [Greek]
Freya	Lady [OldNorse]
Inez	Spanish form of Agnes; pure one [Greek]

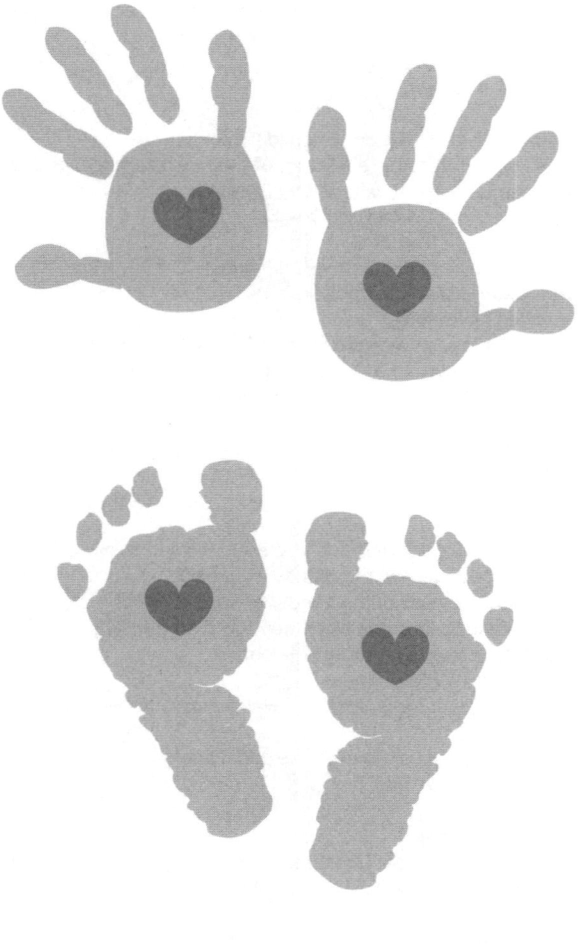

100 Popular *Boys* Names

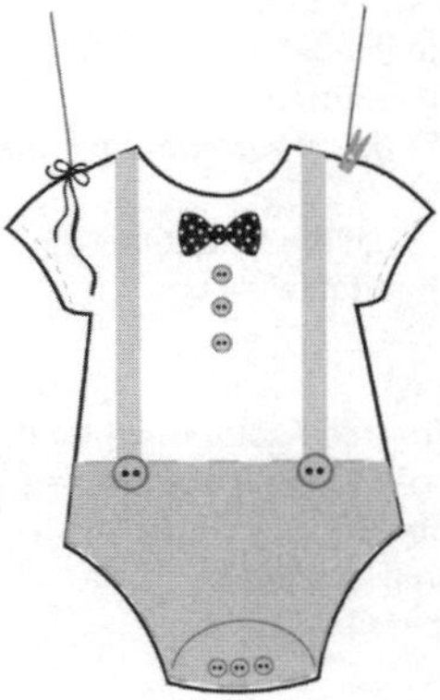

100 Popular Boys Names

Noah	Rest; comfort [Hebrew]
Liam	Irish diminutive of William; resolute protector [Old German]
Oliver	Elf warrior [Old German]; Or ancestor's descendant [Old Norse]
Lucas	Variant of Luke; from Lucania, southern Italy [Greek]
Mason	From the surname; stoneworker [Old German]
Ethan	Firm; enduring [Hebrew]
Aiden	Variant of Aidan; little fire [Gaelic]
Elijah	My God is Jehova [Hebrew]
James	English form of Jacob; supplanter [Hebrew]
Jacob	Holder of the heel; supplanter [Hebrew]
Benjamin	Son of the south; son of the right hand [Hebrew]
Logan	From the Scottish surname; from the little hollow [Gaelic]
Jackson	Son of Jack, a diminutive of John; God is gracious [Hebrew]
Sebastian	From Sebaste, Asia Minor [Latin]
Jack	Diminutive of John; God is gracious [Hebrew]
Alexander	The defender [Greek]
Michael	Who is like God? [Hebrew]
Carter	From the surname; cart user/worker
Jayden	Variant of Jaden; God has heard; judge; thankful [Hebrew]
Matthew	Gift of God [Hebrew]
Luke	From Lucania, southern Italy [Greek]
Grayson	From the surname; son of the steward [Old English]
Wyatt	From the surname; battle brave [Old English]
William	Resolute protector [Old German]
Gabriel	God is my strength [Hebrew]
Daniel	God is my judge [Hebrew]
Henry	Home ruler [Old German]
Owen	Welsh form of Eugene; well-born [Greek]. Or youth [Welsh]
Levi	Joined [Hebrew]
Ryan	From the surname; little king [Gaelic]
Caleb	Dog; or whole heart [Hebrew]
Adam	Man [Hebrew]
David	Beloved [Hebrew]
Lincoln	From Lincoln; from the settlement by the lake, pool [Celtic/Latin]
Muhammad	Turkish variant of Muhammed; praised one; praiseworthy [Arabic]
Joseph	He will add [Hebrew]
Isaiah	God is salvation [Hebew]
Eli	Ascension [Hebrew]
Leo	Lion [Latin]
Samuel	Name of God; God has heard [Hebrew]
Julian	From the Roman name Iulianus/Julius; downy-bearded [Latin]
Josiah	God supports [Hebrew]
Dylan	Great one from the sea [Welsh]
Isaac	He will laugh; he will rejoice [Hebrew]
Joshua	God is salvation [Hebrew]
Andrew	Strong; manly [Greek]
John	God is gracious [Hebrew]
Christian	Christian
Charlie	Diminutive of Charles; man; warrior [Old German]
Cameron	From the Scottish surname; crooked nose [Gaelic]

Hunter	From the surname; hunter
Nathan	He gave [Hebrew]
Anthony	Meaning unknown; possibly priceless; handsome [Etruscan]
Connor	Variant of Conor; dog-lover; wolf-lover [Gaelic]
Christopher	Bearing Christ; carrying Christ [Greek]
Mateo	Sapanish form of Matthew; git of God [Henrew]
Landon	From the surname; from the long hill [Old English]
Jeremiah	God has lifted [Hebrew]
Easton	From the surname; from the east town [Old English]
Brayden	Variant of Braden; from the Irish surname; salmon [Irish]
Asher	Happy; blessed [Hebrew]
Jordan	From the name of the river
Aaron	High; exalted [Hebrew]
Ezra	Help [Hebrew]
Hudson	Son of Hudde, a diminutive of Hugh; heart; spirit [Old German]
Jace	Diminutive of Jason; to heal; healer [Greek]
Nicholas	Victory of the people [Greek]
Xavier	New house [Basque]
Bryson	From the surname; son of Brice; son of the speckled one
Thomas	Twin [Aramaic/Greek]
Evan	Anglicized variant of Iefan, Welsh form of John; God is gracious [Hebrew]
Max	Form of Maximilian; greatest [Latin]. Mack's/Magnus's stream [Old English/Norse]
Nolan	From the Irish surname; noble or famous little one [Irish]
Austin	Contraction of Augustine; great [Latin]
Dominic	Of the Lord [Latin]
Colton	From the surname; from Cola's town; from colt-breeding town
Carson	One from the marsh [Old English]; from the fort [Welsh]; from the rock [Gaelic]
Elias	Variant of Elijah; my God is Jehova [Hebrew]
Kayden	Variant of Caden; spirit of battle [Gaelic]. Or friend; companion [Arabic]
Jaxon	Variant of Jackson; son of Jack, a diminutive of John; God is gracious [Hebrew]
Bentley	From the surname; from the bent grass woodland [Old English]
Gavin	Variant of Gawain; hawk of May [Welsh]
Jonathan	God has given [Hebrew]
Kai	Sea [Hawaian]
Maverick	Maverick; independent
Cooper	From the surname; barrel maker [Old English]
Ezekiel	God strenghens [Hebrew]
Alex	Diminutive of Alexander; the defender [Greek]
George	Farmer [Greek]
Parker	From the surname; park keeper
Tyler	From the surname; roof tiler
King	From a nickname; king; kingly [Old English]
Robert	Bright fame [Old German]
Chase	From the surname; huntsman [Old English]
Santiago	Chilean city, or saint's name; St. James; supplanter [Hebrew]
Luca	Italian variant of Luke; from Lucania, southern Italy [Greek]
Oscar	Deer friend [Gaelic]; or god spear [Old English]
Harry	Diminutive of Henry; home ruler [Old German]
Freddie	Diminutive of Frederick; peaceful ruler [Old German]
Miles	Variant of Milo; gracious [Slavic]; or soldier [Latin]

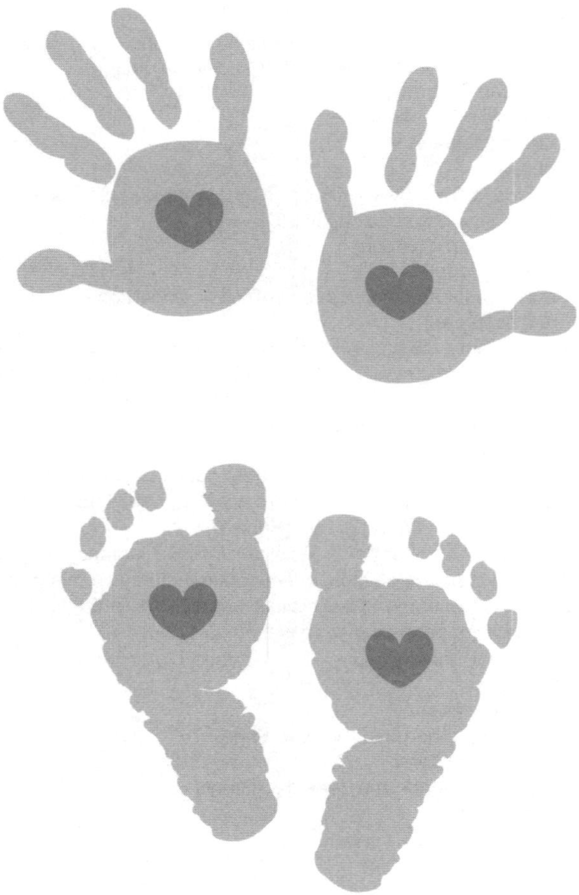